Chronic
Pain & Fatigue

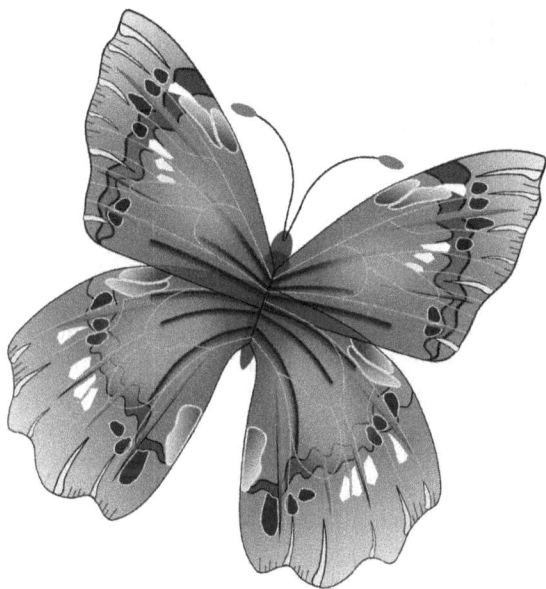

DIARY

C.S. Casey

First published in 2017
© 2017 C.S. Casey.

CME Books
Penrith NSW 2750
Australia
ABN 51 087 646 671

National Library of Australia
Cataloguing-in-Publication entry:
Casey, Char
Chronic Pain & Fatigue Diary

ISBN 13: 978-0-9942137-3-0

Notice of Liability

The author and publisher have made every attempt to provide the reader with accurate, timely, and useful information. The information presented is for reference purposes only. While every precaution has been taken in the preparation of this book, the author and publisher make no claims that using this information will guarantee the reader success and neither the author nor publisher shall have any liability to any person or entity with respect to any liability, loss, or damage caused or alleged to be caused directly or indirectly by the instructions contained in this book or by the computer software products described herein.

Some graphics and textures used in the design of the cover and interior pages of this diary were sourced from the kind folks at *Freepik.com* and *Pixabay.com*

Typesetting & Cover Design by Char Casey

10 9 8 7 6 5 4 3 2 1

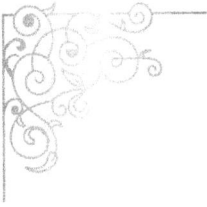

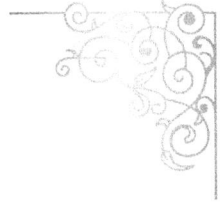

This Pain Diary belongs to

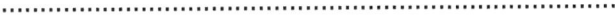

....

If found, please contact me on

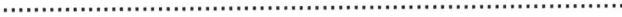

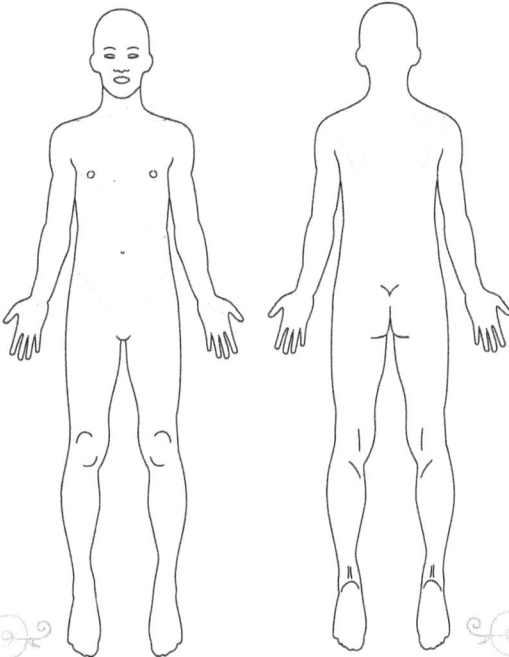

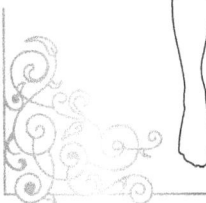

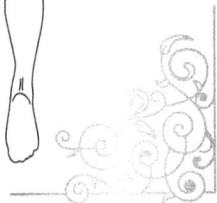

....

Appointments (Consultations, Tests & Treatments)

Date ...... / ...... / ......   Time .... am /pm   With ....

Where ....   Purpose ....

Date ...... / ...... / ......   Time .... am /pm   With ....

Where ....   Purpose ....

Date ...... / ...... / ......   Time .... am /pm   With ....

Where ....   Purpose ....

Date ...... / ...... / ......   Time .... am /pm   With ....

Where ....   Purpose ....

Date ...... / ...... / ......   Time .... am /pm   With ....

Where ....   Purpose ....

Date ...... / ...... / ......   Time .... am /pm   With ....

Where ....   Purpose ....

Date ...... / ...... / ......   Time .... am /pm   With ....

Where ....   Purpose ....

Date ...... / ...... / ......   Time .... am /pm   With ....

Where ....   Purpose ....

Date ...... / ...... / ......   Time .... am /pm   With ....

Where ....   Purpose ....

Date ...... / ...... / ......   Time .... am /pm   With ....

Where ....   Purpose ....

Date ...... / ...... / ......   Time .... am /pm   With ....

Where ....   Purpose ....

Date ...... / ...... / ......   Time .... am /pm   With ....

Where ....   Purpose ....

MONTH
One

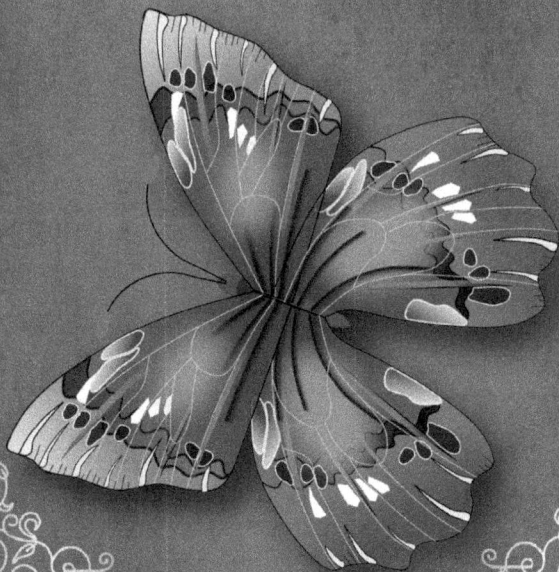

Date: ___ / ___ / ___

Day ___

Sleep

Bed (last night)	_____ am / pm
Asleep	_____ am / pm
Woke up	_____ am / pm
# of Disruptions	_____
Total Hours slept	_____

Medications

☐ No Change in Meds

☐ Dosage Changed

☐ New Medication

Details _____

Today's Ratings

Scale: 0 = None, 10 = Severe

Pain	_____ / 10
Fatigue	_____ / 10
Weakness	_____ / 10
Stiffness	_____ / 10
Anxiety	_____ / 10
Depression	_____ / 10
Stress	_____ / 10
Anger	_____ / 10
Brain Fog / Forgetfulness	_____ / 10

Pain location(s)

Circle or shade in where your pain is using pen, pencil or highlighters

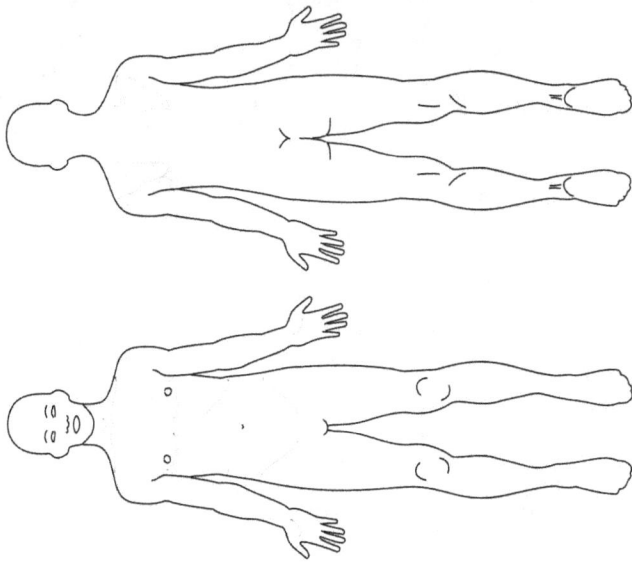

Activity

Active

- [ ] Walking
- [ ] Gym
- [ ] Housework
- [ ] Hydrotherapy

Passive

- [ ] Reading
- [ ] TV
- [ ] Music
- [ ] Light Housework

Meals

Breakfast

Lunch

Dinner

Snacks & Dessert

Beverages

- [ ] Juice
- [ ] Tea
- [ ] Milk
- [ ] Soft D
- [ ] Water
- [ ] Coffee
- [ ] Energy

Symptoms

Date: ___ / ___ / ___   Day ___

Sleep

Bed (last night)	_____ am / pm
Asleep	_____ am / pm
Woke up	_____ am / pm
# of Disruptions	_____
Total Hours slept	_____

Medications

☐ No Change in Meds
☐ Dosage Changed
☐ New Medication

Details _____

_____

Today's Ratings
Scale: 0 = None, 10 = Severe

Pain	___ / 10
Fatigue	___ / 10
Weakness	___ / 10
Stiffness	___ / 10
Anxiety	___ / 10
Depression	___ / 10
Stress	___ / 10
Anger	___ / 10
Brain Fog / Forgetfulness	___ / 10

Pain location(s)
Circle or shade in where your pain is using pen, pencil or highlighters

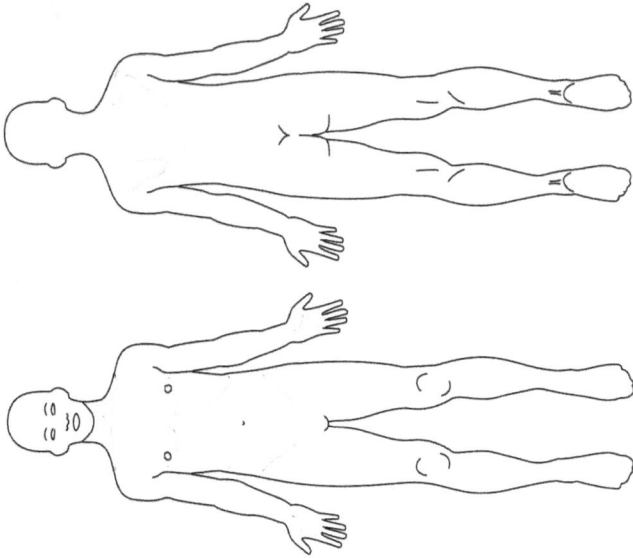

Activity

Active

- ☐ Walking
- ☐ Gym
- ☐ Housework
- ☐ Hydrotherapy

Passive

- ☐ Reading
- ☐ TV
- ☐ Music
- ☐ Light Housework

Meals

Breakfast

Lunch

Dinner

Snacks & Dessert

Beverages

- ☐ Juice
- ☐ Tea
- ☐ Water
- ☐ Milk
- ☐ Soft D
- ☐ Coffee
- ☐ Energy

Symptoms

Date: _____ / _____ / _____   Day _____

Sleep

Bed (last night) _____ am / pm

Asleep _____ am / pm

Woke up _____ am / pm

# of Disruptions _____

Total Hours slept _____

Today's Ratings

Scale: 0 = None, 10 = Severe

Pain	____ / 10
Fatigue	____ / 10
Weakness	____ / 10
Stiffness	____ / 10
Anxiety	____ / 10
Depression	____ / 10
Stress	____ / 10
Anger	____ / 10
Brain Fog / Forgetfulness	____ / 10

Medications

☐ No Change in Meds

☐ Dosage Changed

☐ New Medication

Details _____

Pain location(s)

Circle or shade in where your pain is using pen, pencil or highlighters

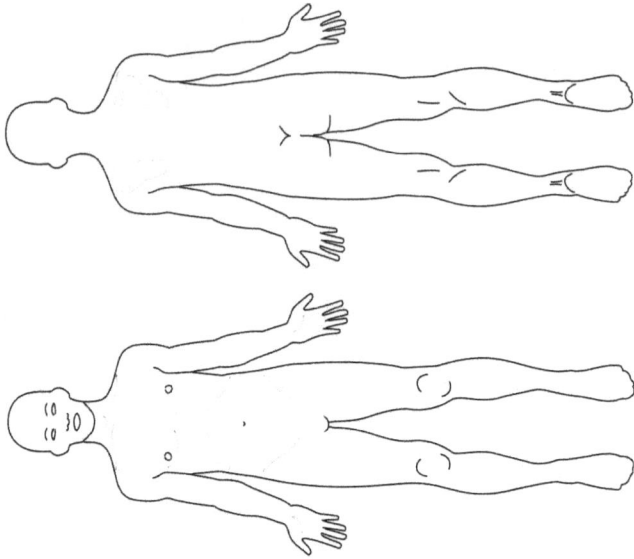

Symptoms

Meals

Breakfast

Lunch

Dinner

Snacks & Dessert

Beverages

- [ ] Juice
- [ ] Milk
- [ ] Tea
- [ ] Soft D
- [ ] Water
- [ ] Coffee
- [ ] Energy

Activity

Active

- [ ] Walking
- [ ] Housework
- [ ] Gym
- [ ] Hydrotherapy

Passive

- [ ] Reading
- [ ] Music
- [ ] TV
- [ ] Light Housework

Date: ____ / ____ / ____   Day ____

Sleep

Bed (last night)	_____ am / pm
Asleep	_____ am / pm
Woke up	_____ am / pm
# of Disruptions	_____
Total Hours slept	_____

Medications

☐ No Change in Meds

☐ Dosage Changed

☐ New Medication

Details _____

_____

Today's Ratings

Scale: 0 = None, 10 = Severe

Pain	_____ / 10
Fatigue	_____ / 10
Weakness	_____ / 10
Stiffness	_____ / 10
Anxiety	_____ / 10
Depression	_____ / 10
Stress	_____ / 10
Anger	_____ / 10
Brain Fog / Forgetfulness	_____ / 10

Pain location(s)

Circle or shade in where your pain is using pen, pencil or highlighters

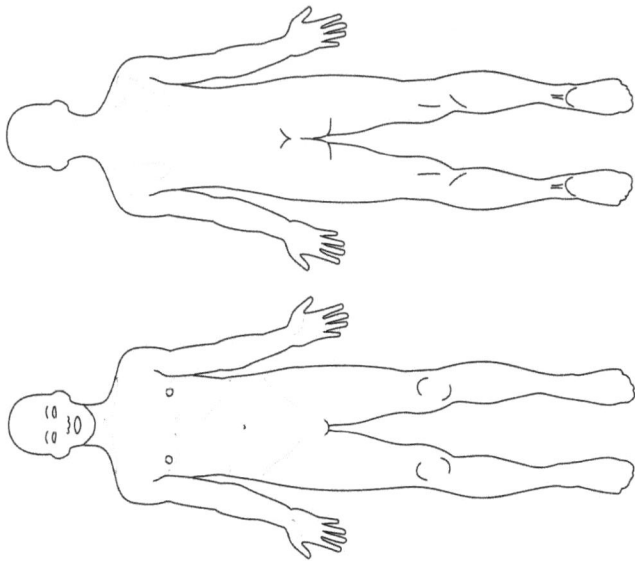

Activity

Active
- [ ] Walking
- [ ] Gym
- [ ] Housework
- [ ] Hydrotherapy

Passive
- [ ] Reading
- [ ] TV
- [ ] Music
- [ ] Light Housework

Meals

Breakfast

Lunch

Dinner

Snacks & Dessert

Beverages
- [ ] Juice
- [ ] Tea
- [ ] Water
- [ ] Milk
- [ ] Soft D
- [ ] Coffee
- [ ] Energy

Symptoms

Date: _____ / _____ / _____   Day _____

Sleep

Bed (last night)	_____ am / pm
Asleep	_____ am / pm
Woke up	_____ am / pm
# of Disruptions	_____
Total Hours slept	_____

Medications

☐ No Change in Meds

☐ Dosage Changed

☐ New Medication

Details _____

_____

Today's Ratings

Scale 0 = None, 10 = Severe

Pain	_____ / 10
Fatigue	_____ / 10
Weakness	_____ / 10
Stiffness	_____ / 10
Anxiety	_____ / 10
Depression	_____ / 10
Stress	_____ / 10
Anger	_____ / 10
Brain Fog / Forgetfulness	_____ / 10

Pain location(s)

Circle or shade in where your pain is using pen, pencil or highlighters

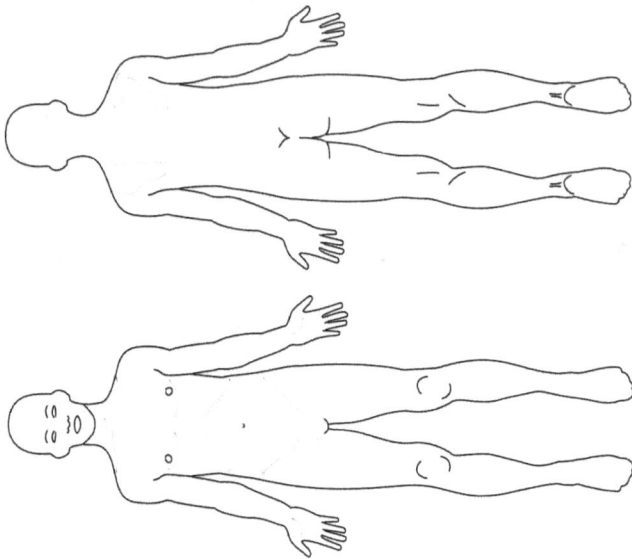

Activity

Active

- [ ] Walking
- [ ] Gym
- [ ] Housework
- [ ] Hydrotherapy

Passive

- [ ] Reading
- [ ] TV
- [ ] Music
- [ ] Light Housework

Meals

Breakfast

Lunch

Dinner

Snacks & Dessert

Beverages

- [ ] Juice
- [ ] Tea
- [ ] Water
- [ ] Milk
- [ ] Soft D
- [ ] Coffee
- [ ] Energy

Symptoms

Date: ___ / ___ / ___

Day ___

Sleep

Bed (last night) ___ am / pm

Asleep ___ am / pm

Woke up ___ am / pm

# of Disruptions ___

Total Hours slept ___

Medications

☐ No Change in Meds

☐ Dosage Changed

☐ New Medication

Details ___

___

Today's Ratings

Scale: 0 = None, 10 = Severe

Pain ___ /10

Fatigue ___ /10

Weakness ___ /10

Stiffness ___ /10

Anxiety ___ /10

Depression ___ /10

Stress ___ /10

Anger ___ /10

Brain Fog / Forgetfulness ___ /10

Pain location(s)

Circle or shade in where your pain is using pen, pencil or highlighters

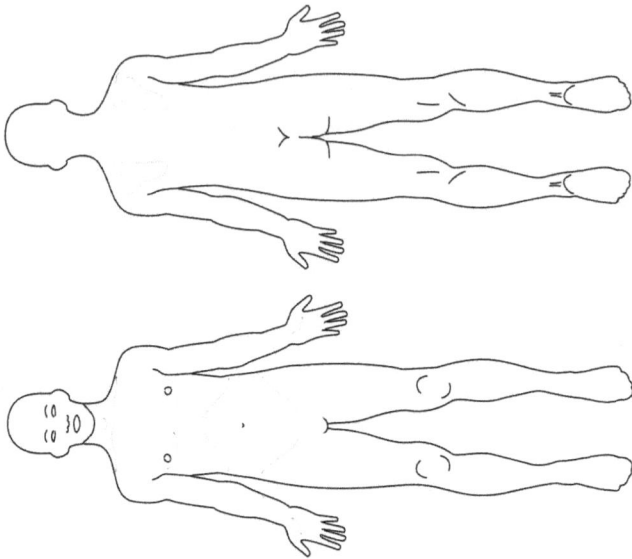

Activity

Active

- [ ] Walking
- [ ] Housework
- [ ] Gym
- [ ] Hydrotherapy

Passive

- [ ] Reading
- [ ] Music
- [ ] TV
- [ ] Light Housework

Meals

Breakfast

Lunch

Dinner

Snacks & Dessert

Beverages

- [ ] Juice
- [ ] Milk
- [ ] Tea
- [ ] Soft D
- [ ] Water
- [ ] Coffee
- [ ] Energy

Symptoms

Date: ___ / ___ / ___   Day ___

Sleep

Bed (last night)	_____ am / pm
Asleep	_____ am / pm
Woke up	_____ am / pm
# of Disruptions	_____
Total/Hours slept	

Medications

☐ No Change in Meds

☐ Dosage Changed

☐ New Medication

Details

Today's Ratings
Scale: 0 = None, 10 = Severe

Pain	_____ / 10
Fatigue	_____ / 10
Weakness	_____ / 10
Stiffness	_____ / 10
Anxiety	_____ / 10
Depression	_____ / 10
Stress	_____ / 10
Anger	_____ / 10
Brain Fog / Forgetfulness	_____ / 10

Pain location(s)

Circle or shade in where your pain is using pen, pencil or highlighters

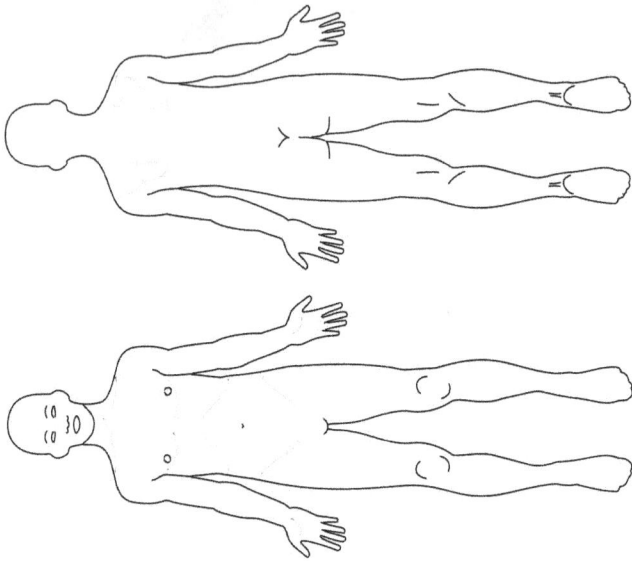

Activity

Active

- [ ] Walking
- [ ] Gym
- [ ] Housework
- [ ] Hydrotherapy

Passive

- [ ] Reading
- [ ] TV
- [ ] Music
- [ ] Light Housework

Meals

Breakfast

Lunch

Dinner

Snacks & Dessert

Beverages

- [ ] Juice
- [ ] Tea
- [ ] Water
- [ ] Milk
- [ ] Soft D
- [ ] Coffee
- [ ] Energy

Symptoms

Date: ____ / ____ / ____   Day ____

Sleep

Bed (last night) _____ am / pm

Asleep _____ am / pm

Woke up _____ am / pm

# of Disruptions _____

Total/Hours slept _____

Medications

☐ No Change in Meds

☐ Dosage Changed

☐ New Medication

Details _____

Today's Ratings

Scale: 0 = None, 10 = Severe

Pain _____ / 10

Fatigue _____ / 10

Weakness _____ / 10

Stiffness _____ / 10

Anxiety _____ / 10

Depression _____ / 10

Stress _____ / 10

Anger _____ / 10

Brain Fog / _____ / 10
Forgetfulness

Pain location(s)

Circle or shade in where your pain is using pen, pencil or highlighters

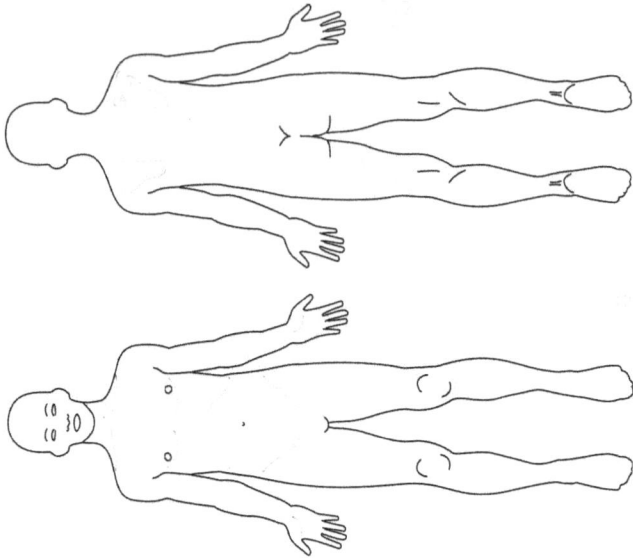

Activity

Active

☐ Walking ☐ Gym
☐ Housework ☐ Hydrotherapy

Passive

☐ Reading ☐ TV
☐ Music ☐ Light Housework

Meals

Breakfast

Lunch

Dinner

Snacks & Dessert

Beverages

☐ Juice ☐ Tea ☐ Water
☐ Milk ☐ Soft D ☐ Coffee
☐ Energy

Symptoms

Date: ___ / ___ / ___   Day ___

Sleep

Bed (last night) _____ am / pm

Asleep _____ am / pm

Woke up _____ am / pm

# of Disruptions _____

Total Hours slept _____

Medications

☐ No Change in Meds

☐ Dosage Changed

☐ New Medication

Details

Today's Ratings

Scale: 0 = None, 10 = Severe

Pain _____ / 10

Fatigue _____ / 10

Weakness _____ / 10

Stiffness _____ / 10

Anxiety _____ / 10

Depression _____ / 10

Stress _____ / 10

Anger _____ / 10

Brain Fog / _____ / 10
Forgetfulness

Pain location(s)

Circle or shade in where your pain is using pen, pencil or highlighters

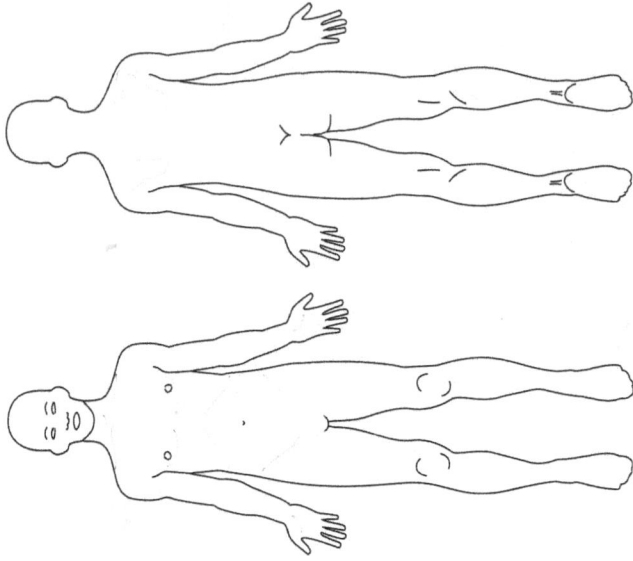

Symptoms

Meals

Breakfast

Lunch

Dinner

Snacks & Dessert

Beverages

☐ Juice ☐ Tea ☐ Water

☐ Milk ☐ Soft D ☐ Coffee

☐ Energy

Activity

Active

☐ Walking ☐ Gym

☐ Housework ☐ Hydrotherapy

Passive

☐ Reading ☐ TV

☐ Music ☐ Light Housework

Date: ___ / ___ / ___   Day ___

Sleep

Bed (last night)	_____ am / pm
Asleep	_____ am / pm
Woke up	_____ am / pm
# of Disruptions	_____
Total Hours slept	_____

Medications

☐ No Change in Meds
☐ Dosage Changed
☐ New Medication

Details _____

Today's Ratings

Scale: 0 = None, 10 = Severe

Pain	___ /10
Fatigue	___ /10
Weakness	___ /10
Stiffness	___ /10
Anxiety	___ /10
Depression	___ /10
Stress	___ /10
Anger	___ /10
Brain Fog / Forgetfulness	___ /10

Pain location(s)

Circle or shade in where your pain is using pen, pencil or highlighters

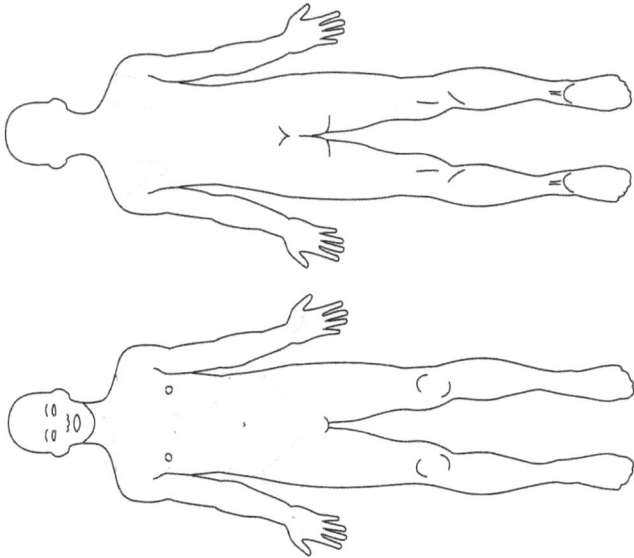

Symptoms

Meals

Breakfast

Lunch

Dinner

Snacks & Dessert

Beverages

☐ Juice ☐ Tea ☐ Water

☐ Milk ☐ Soft D ☐ Coffee

☐ Energy

Activity

Active

☐ Walking ☐ Gym

☐ Housework ☐ Hydrotherapy

Passive

☐ Reading ☐ TV

☐ Music ☐ Light Housework

Date: ___ / ___ / ___

Day ___

Sleep

Bed (last night)	___ am / pm
Asleep	___ am / pm
Woke up	___ am / pm
# of Disruptions	___
Total Hours slept	___

Medications

☐ No Change in Meds

☐ Dosage Changed

☐ New Medication

Details

Today's Ratings

Scale: 0 = None, 10 = Severe

Pain	___ / 10
Fatigue	___ / 10
Weakness	___ / 10
Stiffness	___ / 10
Anxiety	___ / 10
Depression	___ / 10
Stress	___ / 10
Anger	___ / 10
Brain Fog / Forgetfulness	___ / 10

Pain location(s)

Circle or shade in where your pain is using pen, pencil or highlighters

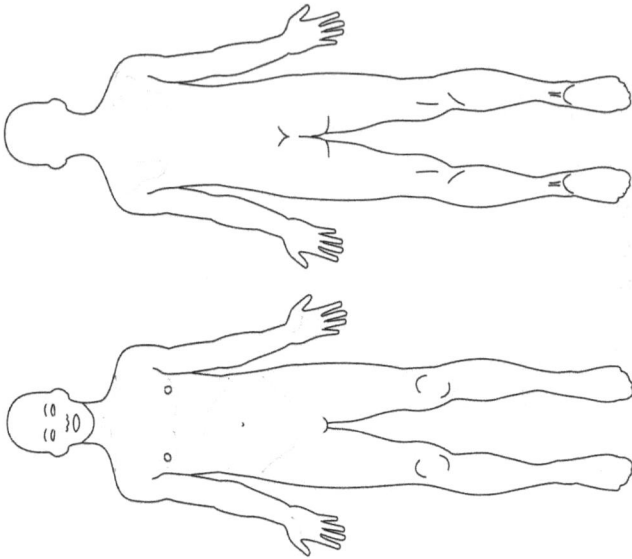

Symptoms

Meals

Breakfast

Lunch

Dinner

Snacks & Dessert

Beverages

- [ ] Juice
- [ ] Milk
- [ ] Tea
- [ ] Soft D
- [ ] Water
- [ ] Coffee
- [ ] Energy

Activity

Active

- [ ] Walking
- [ ] Housework
- [ ] Gym
- [ ] Hydrotherapy

Passive

- [ ] Reading
- [ ] Music
- [ ] TV
- [ ] Light Housework

Date: _____ / ___ / ___

Day ___

Sleep

Bed (last night) _____ am / pm

Asleep _____ am / pm

Woke up _____ am / pm

# of Disruptions _____

Total Hours slept _____

Medications

☐ No Change in Meds

☐ Dosage Changed

☐ New Medication

Details _____

_____

Today's Ratings

Scale: 0 = None, 10 = Severe

Pain _____ / 10

Fatigue _____ / 10

Weakness _____ / 10

Stiffness _____ / 10

Anxiety _____ / 10

Depression _____ / 10

Stress _____ / 10

Anger _____ / 10

Brain Fog / Forgetfulness _____ / 10

Pain location(s)

Circle or shade in where your pain is using pen, pencil or highlighters

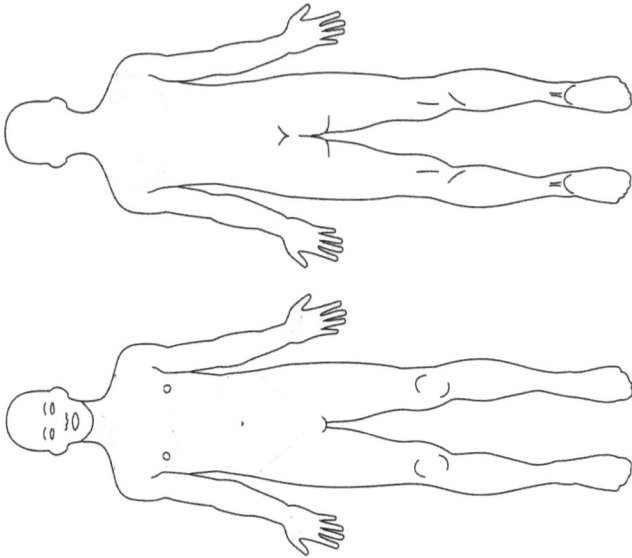

Symptoms

Meals

Breakfast

Lunch

Dinner

Snacks & Dessert

Beverages

☐ Juice ☐ Tea ☐ Water

☐ Milk ☐ Soft D ☐ Coffee

☐ Energy

Activity

Active

☐ Walking ☐ Gym

☐ Housework ☐ Hydrotherapy

Passive

☐ Reading ☐ TV

☐ Music ☐ Light Housework

Date: ___ / ___ / ___

Sleep

Bed (last night)	_____ am / pm
Asleep	_____ am / pm
Woke up	_____ am / pm
# of Disruptions	_____
Total/Hours slept	_____

Medications

☐ No Change in Meds
☐ Dosage Changed
☐ New Medication

Details

_____

Today's Ratings

Scale: 0 = None, 10 = Severe

Pain	_____ / 10
Fatigue	_____ / 10
Weakness	_____ / 10
Stiffness	_____ / 10
Anxiety	_____ / 10
Depression	_____ / 10
Stress	_____ / 10
Anger	_____ / 10
Brain Fog / Forgetfulness	_____ / 10

Day ___

Pain location(s)

Circle or shade in where your pain is using pen, pencil or highlighters

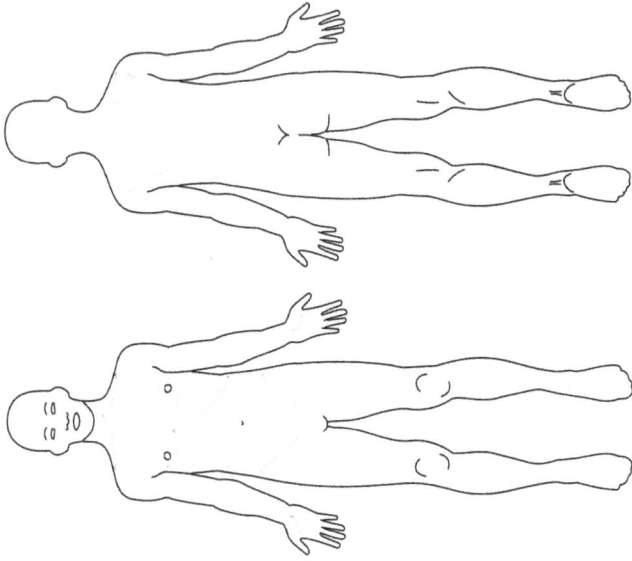

Symptoms

Meals

Breakfast

Lunch

Dinner

Snacks & Dessert

Beverages

- [ ] Juice
- [ ] Tea
- [ ] Milk
- [ ] Soft D
- [ ] Water
- [ ] Coffee
- [ ] Energy

Activity

Active

- [ ] Walking
- [ ] Gym
- [ ] Housework
- [ ] Hydrotherapy

Passive

- [ ] Reading
- [ ] TV
- [ ] Music
- [ ] Light Housework

Date: ___ / ___ / ___   Day ___

Sleep

Bed (last night)	___ am / pm
Asleep	___ am / pm
Woke up	___ am / pm
# of Disruptions	___
Total Hours slept	___

Medications

☐ No Change in Meds

☐ Dosage Changed

☐ New Medication

Details

Today's Ratings

Scale: 0 = None, 10 = Severe

Pain	___ / 10
Fatigue	___ / 10
Weakness	___ / 10
Stiffness	___ / 10
Anxiety	___ / 10
Depression	___ / 10
Stress	___ / 10
Anger	___ / 10
Brain Fog /	___ / 10
Forgetfulness	

Pain location(s)

Circle or shade in where your pain is using pen, pencil or highlighters

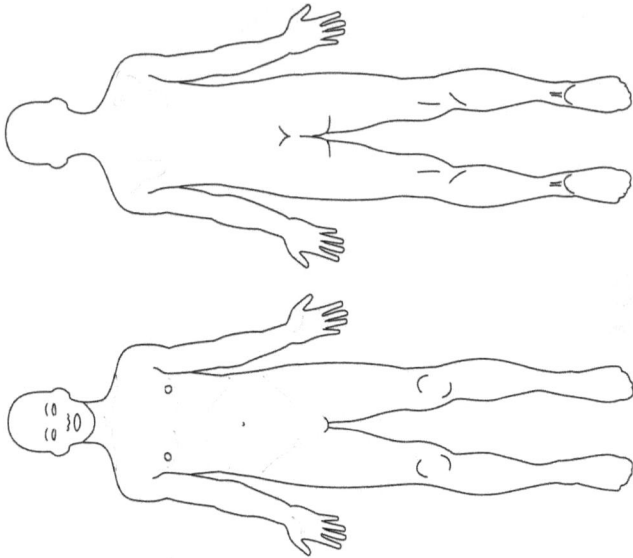

Symptoms

Meals

Breakfast

Lunch

Dinner

Snacks & Dessert

Beverages

☐ Juice ☐ Tea ☐ Water
☐ Milk ☐ Soft D ☐ Coffee
☐ Energy

Activity

Active

☐ Walking ☐ Gym
☐ Housework ☐ Hydrotherapy

Passive

☐ Reading ☐ TV
☐ Music ☐ Light Housework

Date: _____ / _____ / _____

Day _____

Sleep

Bed (last night) _____ am / pm

Asleep _____ am / pm

Woke up _____ am / pm

# of Disruptions _____

Total Hours slept _____

Medications

☐ No Change in Meds

☐ Dosage Changed

☐ New Medication

Details _____

_____

Today's Ratings

Scale: 0 = None, 10 = Severe

Pain _____ / 10

Fatigue _____ / 10

Weakness _____ / 10

Stiffness _____ / 10

Anxiety _____ / 10

Depression _____ / 10

Stress _____ / 10

Anger _____ / 10

Brain Fog / _____ / 10
Forgetfulness

Pain location(s)

Circle or shade in where your pain is using pen, pencil or highlighters

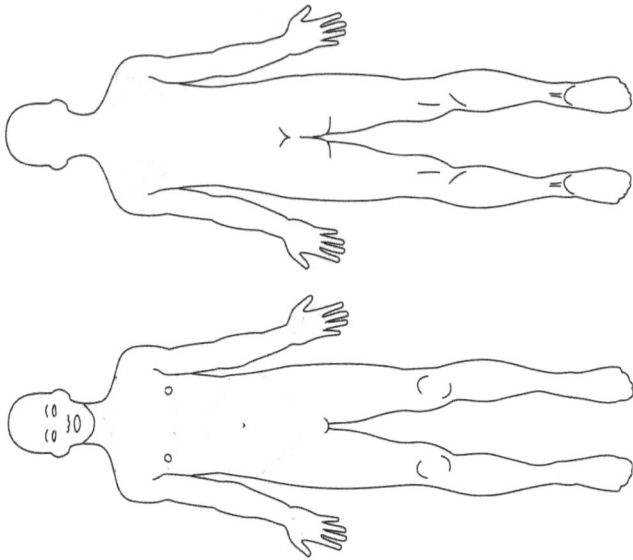

Symptoms

Meals

Breakfast

Lunch

Dinner

Snacks & Dessert

Beverages

☐ Juice ☐ Tea ☐ Water

☐ Milk ☐ Soft D ☐ Coffee

☐ Energy

Activity

Active

☐ Walking ☐ Gym

☐ Housework ☐ Hydrotherapy

Passive

☐ Reading ☐ TV

☐ Music ☐ Light Housework

Date: ___ / ___ / ___

Day____

Sleep

Bed (last night)	____ am / pm
Asleep	____ am / pm
Woke up	____ am / pm
# of Disruptions	____
Total Hours slept	____

Today's Ratings

Scale: 0 = None, 10 = Severe

Pain	____ /10
Fatigue	____ /10
Weakness	____ /10
Stiffness	____ /10
Anxiety	____ /10
Depression	____ /10
Stress	____ /10
Anger	____ /10
Brain Fog / Forgetfulness	____ /10

Medications

☐ No Change in Meds

☐ Dosage Changed

☐ New Medication

Details

Pain location(s)

Circle or shade in where your pain is using pen, pencil or highlighters

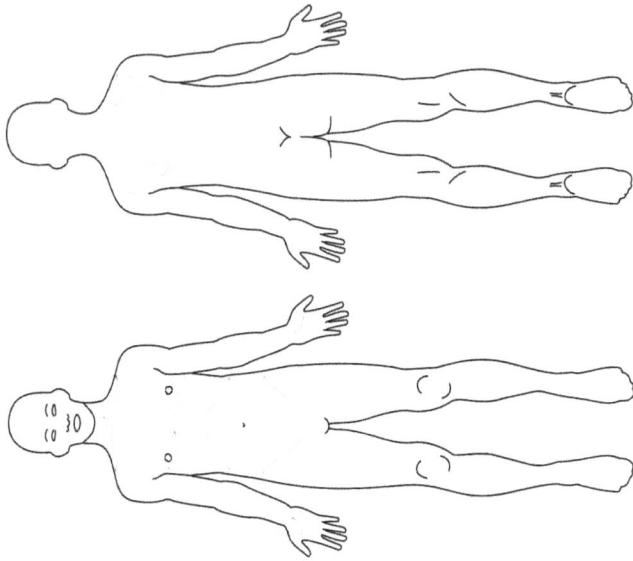

Symptoms

Meals

Breakfast

Lunch

Dinner

Snacks & Dessert

Beverages

☐ Juice ☐ Tea ☐ Water

☐ Milk ☐ Soft D ☐ Coffee

☐ Energy

Activity

Active

☐ Walking ☐ Gym

☐ Housework ☐ Hydrotherapy

Passive

☐ Reading ☐ TV

☐ Music ☐ Light Housework

Date: ___ / ___ / ___   Day ___

Sleep

Bed (last night)	___ am / pm
Asleep	___ am / pm
Woke up	___ am / pm
# of Disruptions	___
Total Hours slept	___

Medications

☐ No Change in Meds

☐ Dosage Changed

☐ New Medication

Details

Today's Ratings

Scale: 0 = None, 10 = Severe

Pain	___ /10
Fatigue	___ /10
Weakness	___ /10
Stiffness	___ /10
Anxiety	___ /10
Depression	___ /10
Stress	___ /10
Anger	___ /10
Brain Fog / Forgetfulness	___ /10

Pain location(s)

Circle or shade in where your pain is using pen, pencil or highlighters

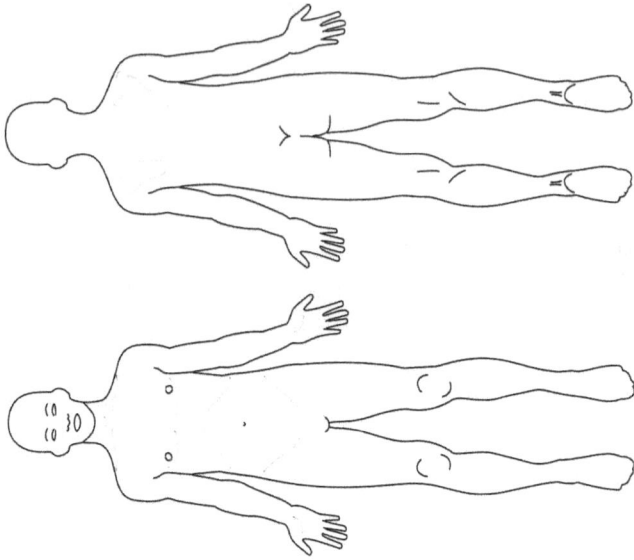

Activity

Active

- [ ] Walking
- [ ] Gym
- [ ] Housework
- [ ] Hydrotherapy

Passive

- [ ] Reading
- [ ] TV
- [ ] Music
- [ ] Light Housework

Meals

Breakfast

Lunch

Dinner

Snacks & Dessert

Beverages

- [ ] Juice
- [ ] Tea
- [ ] Water
- [ ] Milk
- [ ] Soft D
- [ ] Coffee
- [ ] Energy

Symptoms

Date: _____ / _____ / _____

Sleep

Bed (last night)	_____ am / pm
Asleep	_____ am / pm
Woke up	_____ am / pm
# of Disruptions	_____
Total Hours slept	_____

Medications

☐ No Change in Meds

☐ Dosage Changed

☐ New Medication

Details _____

_____

Today's Ratings

Scale: 0 = None, 10 = Severe

Pain	_____ / 10
Fatigue	_____ / 10
Weakness	_____ / 10
Stiffness	_____ / 10
Anxiety	_____ / 10
Depression	_____ / 10
Stress	_____ / 10
Anger	_____ / 10
Brain Fog / Forgetfulness	_____ / 10

Day _____

Pain location(s)

Circle or shade in where your pain is using pen, pencil or highlighters

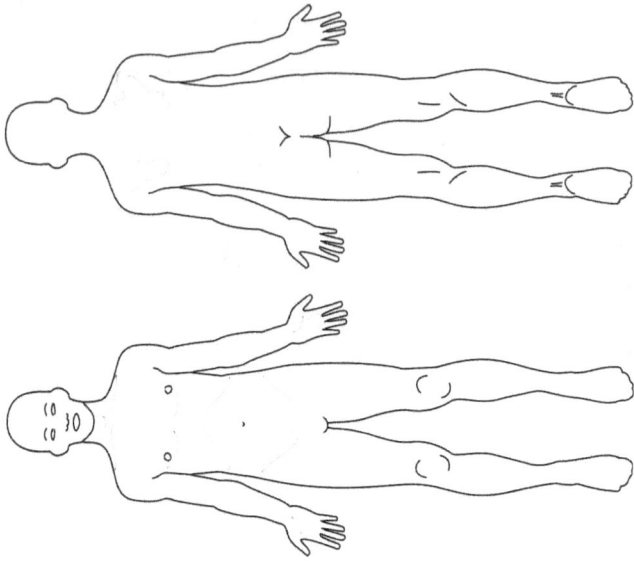

Activity

Active

☐ Walking ☐ Gym
☐ Housework ☐ Hydrotherapy

Passive

☐ Reading ☐ TV
☐ Music ☐ Light Housework

Meals

Breakfast

Lunch

Dinner

Snacks & Dessert

Beverages

☐ Juice ☐ Tea ☐ Water
☐ Milk ☐ Soft D ☐ Coffee
☐ Energy

Symptoms

Date: ___ / ___ / ___

Day ____

Sleep

Bed (last night)	____ am / pm
Asleep	____ am / pm
Woke up	____ am / pm
# of Disruptions	____
Total Hours slept	____

Medications

☐ No Change in Meds

☐ Dosage Changed

☐ New Medication

Details

Today's Ratings

Scale: 0 = None, 10 = Severe

Pain	____ / 10
Fatigue	____ / 10
Weakness	____ / 10
Stiffness	____ / 10
Anxiety	____ / 10
Depression	____ / 10
Stress	____ / 10
Anger	____ / 10
Brain Fog / Forgetfulness	____ / 10

Pain location(s)

Circle or shade in where your pain is using pen, pencil or highlighters

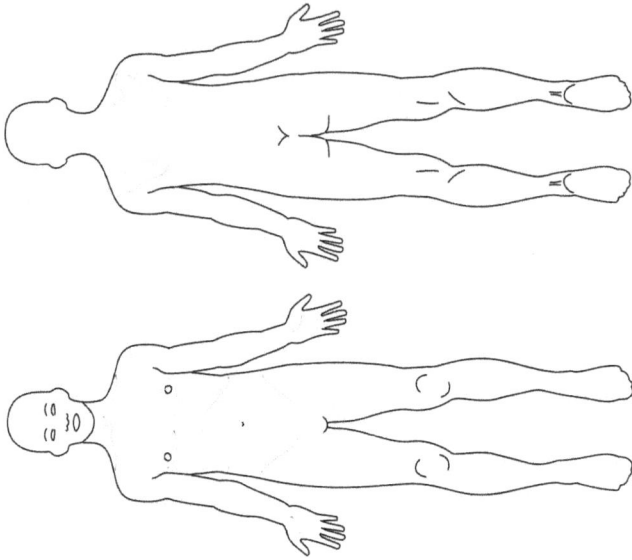

Activity

Active

- [ ] Walking
- [ ] Gym
- [ ] Housework
- [ ] Hydrotherapy

Passive

- [ ] Reading
- [ ] TV
- [ ] Music
- [ ] Light Housework

Meals

Breakfast

Lunch

Dinner

Snacks & Dessert

Beverages

- [ ] Water
- [ ] Coffee
- [ ] Energy
- [ ] Juice
- [ ] Tea
- [ ] Milk
- [ ] Soft D

Symptoms

Date: _____ / _____ / _____

Day _____

Sleep

Bed (last night)	_____ am / pm
Asleep	_____ am / pm
Woke up	_____ am / pm
# of Disruptions	_____
Total Hours slept	_____

Today's Ratings
Scale: 0 = None, 10 = Severe

Pain	_____ / 10
Fatigue	_____ / 10
Weakness	_____ / 10
Stiffness	_____ / 10
Anxiety	_____ / 10
Depression	_____ / 10
Stress	_____ / 10
Anger	_____ / 10
Brain Fog / Forgetfulness	_____ / 10

Medications

☐ No Change in Meds

☐ Dosage Changed

☐ New Medication

Details
_____
_____

Pain location(s)
Circle or shade in where your pain is using pen, pencil or highlighters

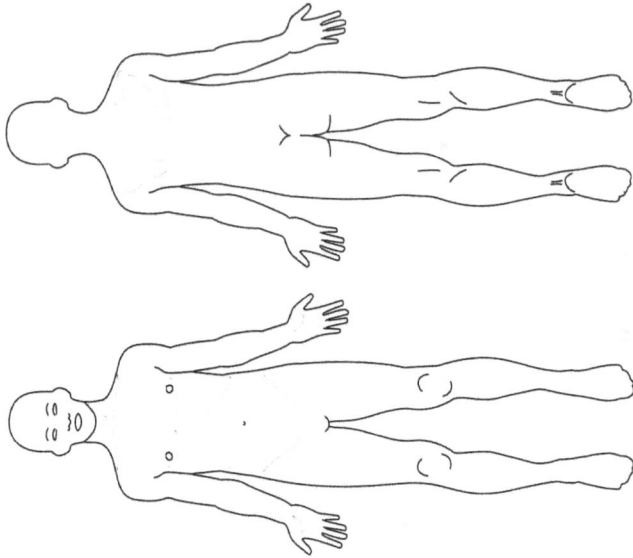

Activity

Active

☐ Walking ☐ Gym
☐ Housework ☐ Hydrotherapy

Passive

☐ Reading ☐ TV
☐ Music ☐ Light Housework

Meals

Breakfast

Lunch

Dinner

Snacks & Dessert

Beverages

☐ Juice ☐ Tea ☐ Water
☐ Milk ☐ Soft D ☐ Coffee
  ☐ Energy

Symptoms

Date: ____ / ____ / ____

Day ____

Sleep

Bed (last night)	_____	am / pm
Asleep	_____	am / pm
Woke up	_____	am / pm
# of Disruptions	_____	
Total Hours slept	_____	

Medications

☐ No Change in Meds

☐ Dosage Changed

☐ New Medication

Details _____

Today's Ratings

Scale: 0 = None, 10 = Severe

Pain	_____ / 10
Fatigue	_____ / 10
Weakness	_____ / 10
Stiffness	_____ / 10
Anxiety	_____ / 10
Depression	_____ / 10
Stress	_____ / 10
Anger	_____ / 10
Brain Fog / Forgetfulness	_____ / 10

Pain location(s)

Circle or shade in where your pain is using pen, pencil or highlighters

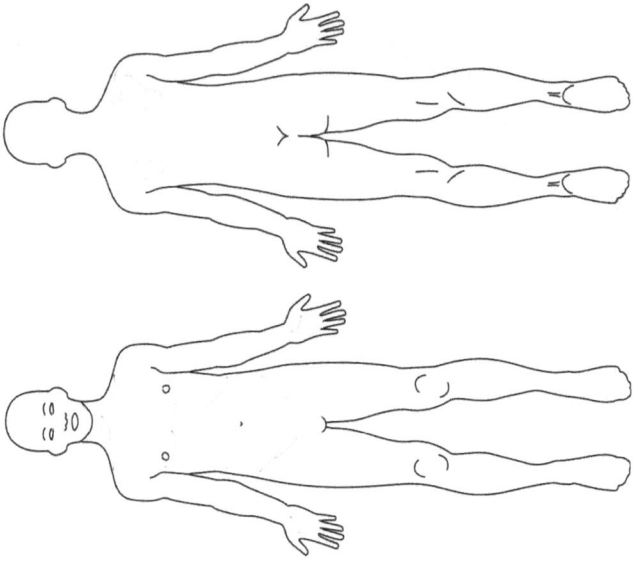

Symptoms

Meals

Breakfast

Lunch

Dinner

Snacks & Dessert

Beverages

- [ ] Juice
- [ ] Milk
- [ ] Tea
- [ ] Soft D
- [ ] Water
- [ ] Coffee
- [ ] Energy

Activity

Active

- [ ] Walking
- [ ] Housework
- [ ] Gym
- [ ] Hydrotherapy

Passive

- [ ] Reading
- [ ] Music
- [ ] TV
- [ ] Light Housework

Date: ___ / ___ / ___   Day ___

Sleep

Bed (last night)	_____ am / pm
Asleep	_____ am / pm
Woke up	_____ am / pm
# of Disruptions	_____
Total Hours slept	_____

Medications

☐ No Change in Meds
☐ Dosage Changed
☐ New Medication

Details _____

Today's Ratings

Scale: 0 = None, 10 = Severe

Pain	_____ / 10
Fatigue	_____ / 10
Weakness	_____ / 10
Stiffness	_____ / 10
Anxiety	_____ / 10
Depression	_____ / 10
Stress	_____ / 10
Anger	_____ / 10
Brain Fog / Forgetfulness	_____ / 10

Pain location(s)

Circle or shade in where your pain is using pen, pencil or highlighters

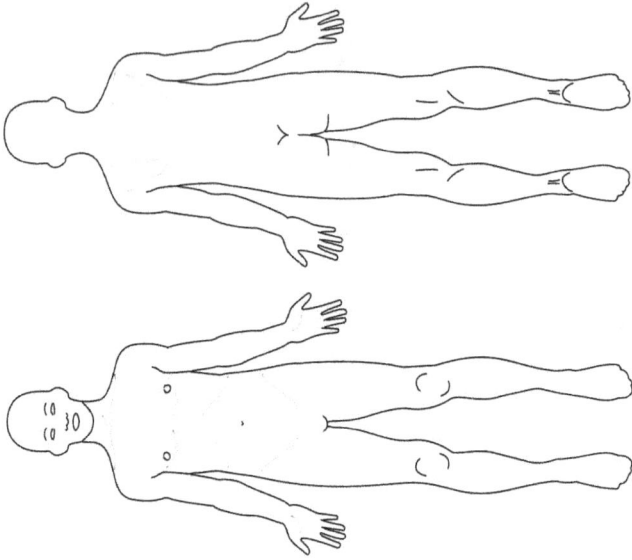

Symptoms

Meals

Breakfast

Lunch

Dinner

Snacks & Dessert

Beverages

☐ Juice ☐ Tea ☐ Water
☐ Milk ☐ Soft D ☐ Coffee
         ☐ Energy

Activity

Active

☐ Walking ☐ Gym
☐ Housework ☐ Hydrotherapy

Passive

☐ Reading ☐ TV
☐ Music ☐ Light Housework

Date: ____ / ____ / ____   Day ____

Sleep

Bed (last night)	____ am / pm
Asleep	____ am / pm
Woke up	____ am / pm
# of Disruptions	____
Total/Hours slept	____

Medications

☐ No Change in Meds

☐ Dosage Changed

☐ New Medication

Details _____

_____

Today's Ratings

Scale: 0 = None, 10 = Severe

Pain	____ / 10
Fatigue	____ / 10
Weakness	____ / 10
Stiffness	____ / 10
Anxiety	____ / 10
Depression	____ / 10
Stress	____ / 10
Anger	____ / 10
Brain Fog / Forgetfulness	____ / 10

Pain location(s)

Circle or shade in where your pain is using pen, pencil or highlighters

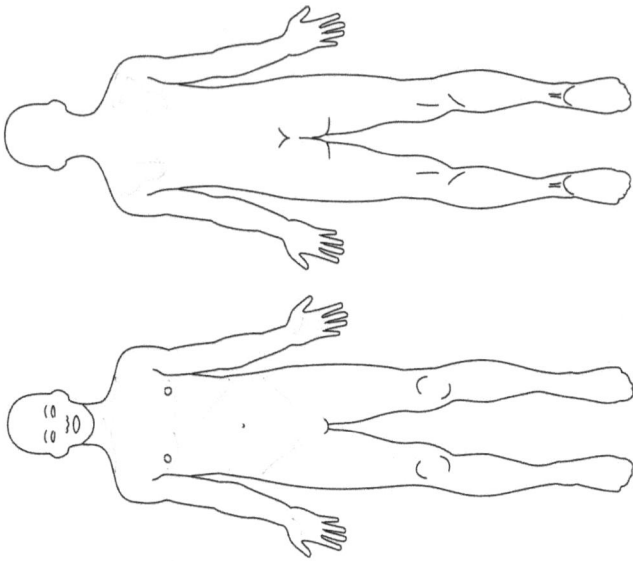

Activity

Active

☐ Walking ☐ Gym
☐ Housework ☐ Hydrotherapy

Passive

☐ Reading ☐ TV
☐ Music ☐ Light Housework

Meals

Breakfast

Lunch

Dinner

Snacks & Dessert

Beverages

☐ Juice ☐ Tea ☐ Water
☐ Milk ☐ Soft D ☐ Coffee
☐ Energy

Symptoms

Date: _____ / _____ / _____

Day _____

Sleep

Bed (last night)	_____ am / pm
Asleep	_____ am / pm
Woke up	_____ am / pm
# of Disruptions	_____
Total Hours slept	_____

Medications

☐ No Change in Meds

☐ Dosage Changed

☐ New Medication

Details _____

_____

Today's Ratings

Scale: 0 = None, 10 = Severe

Pain	_____ / 10
Fatigue	_____ / 10
Weakness	_____ / 10
Stiffness	_____ / 10
Anxiety	_____ / 10
Depression	_____ / 10
Stress	_____ / 10
Anger	_____ / 10
Brain Fog / Forgetfulness	_____ / 10

Pain location(s)

Circle or shade in where your pain is using pen, pencil or highlighters

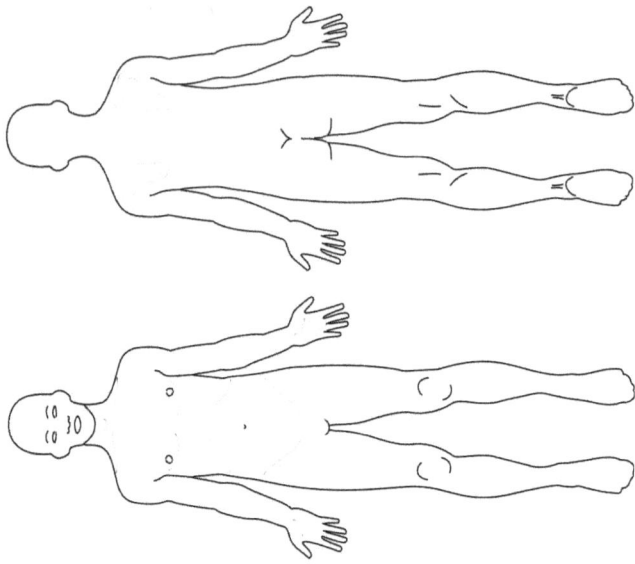

Activity

Active

- [ ] Walking
- [ ] Gym
- [ ] Housework
- [ ] Hydrotherapy

Passive

- [ ] Reading
- [ ] TV
- [ ] Music
- [ ] Light Housework

Meals

Breakfast

Lunch

Dinner

Snacks & Dessert

Beverages

- [ ] Juice
- [ ] Tea
- [ ] Water
- [ ] Milk
- [ ] Soft D
- [ ] Coffee
- [ ] Energy

Symptoms

Date: ___ / ___ / ___

Day ___

Sleep

Bed (last night)	_____ am / pm
Asleep	_____ am / pm
Woke up	_____ am / pm
# of Disruptions	_____
Total Hours slept	_____

Medications

☐ No Change in Meds

☐ Dosage Changed

☐ New Medication

Details _____

_____

Today's Ratings

Scale: 0 = None, 10 = Severe

Pain	___ / 10
Fatigue	___ / 10
Weakness	___ / 10
Stiffness	___ / 10
Anxiety	___ / 10
Depression	___ / 10
Stress	___ / 10
Anger	___ / 10
Brain Fog / Forgetfulness	___ / 10

Pain location(s)

Circle or shade in where your pain is using pen, pencil or highlighters

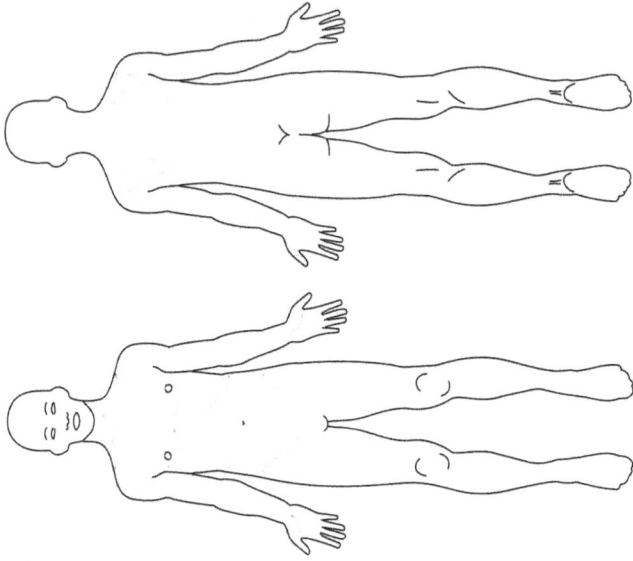

Activity

Active

☐ Walking ☐ Gym
☐ Housework ☐ Hydrotherapy

Passive

☐ Reading ☐ TV
☐ Music ☐ Light Housework

Meals

Breakfast

Lunch

Dinner

Snacks & Dessert

Beverages

☐ Juice ☐ Tea ☐ Water
☐ Milk ☐ Soft D ☐ Coffee
☐ Energy

Symptoms

Date: _____ / _____ / _____

Day _____

Sleep

Bed (last night)	_____ am / pm
Asleep	_____ am / pm
Woke up	_____ am / pm
# of Disruptions	_____
Total Hours slept	_____

Medications

☐ No Change in Meds

☐ Dosage Changed

☐ New Medication

Details _____

Today's Ratings

Scale: 0 = None, 10 = Severe

Pain	_____ / 10
Fatigue	_____ / 10
Weakness	_____ / 10
Stiffness	_____ / 10
Anxiety	_____ / 10
Depression	_____ / 10
Stress	_____ / 10
Anger	_____ / 10
Brain Fog / Forgetfulness	_____ / 10

Pain location(s)

Circle or shade in where your pain is using pen, pencil or highlighters

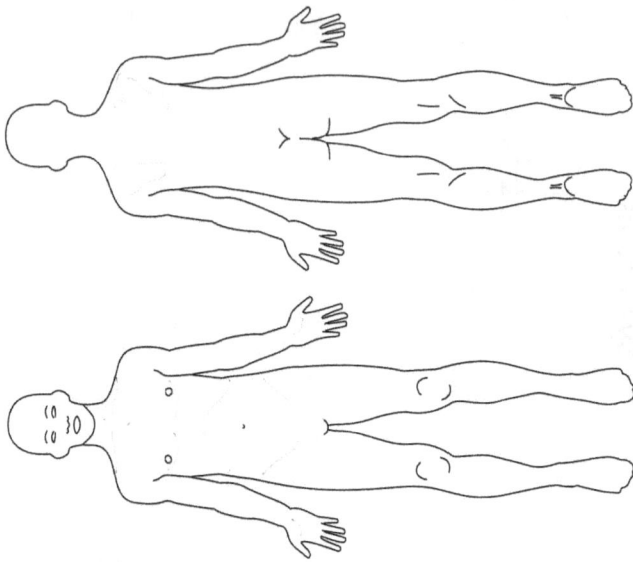

Symptoms

Meals

Breakfast

Lunch

Dinner

Snacks & Dessert

Beverages

☐ Juice ☐ Tea ☐ Water
☐ Milk ☐ Soft D ☐ Coffee
         ☐ Energy

Activity

Active

☐ Walking ☐ Gym
☐ Housework ☐ Hydrotherapy

Passive

☐ Reading ☐ TV
☐ Music ☐ Light Housework

Date: ___ / ___ / ___

Day ___

Sleep

Bed (last night)	___ am / pm
Asleep	___ am / pm
Woke up	___ am / pm
# of Disruptions	___
Total Hours slept	___

Medications

☐ No Change in Meds

☐ Dosage Changed

☐ New Medication

Details _____

_____

Today's Ratings

Scale: 0 = None, 10 = Severe

Pain	___ /10
Fatigue	___ /10
Weakness	___ /10
Stiffness	___ /10
Anxiety	___ /10
Depression	___ /10
Stress	___ /10
Anger	___ /10
Brain Fog / Forgetfulness	___ /10

Pain location(s)

Circle or shade in where your pain is using pen, pencil or highlighters

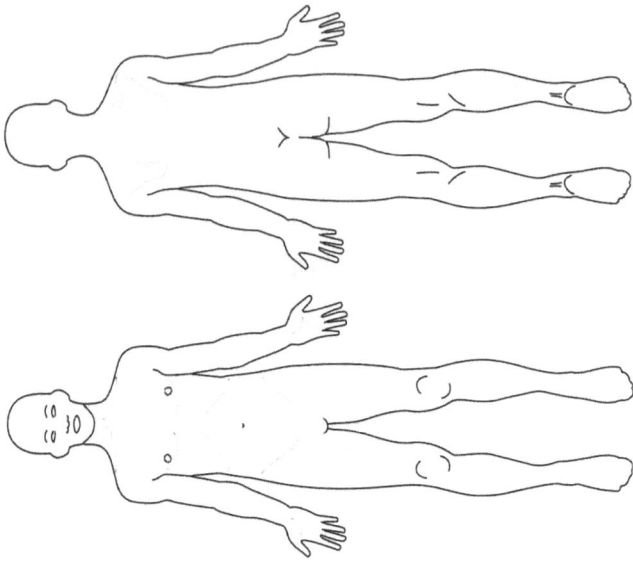

Symptoms

Meals

Breakfast

Lunch

Dinner

Snacks & Dessert

Beverages

- [ ] Juice
- [ ] Milk
- [ ] Tea
- [ ] Soft D
- [ ] Water
- [ ] Coffee
- [ ] Energy

Activity

Active

- [ ] Walking
- [ ] Housework
- [ ] Gym
- [ ] Hydrotherapy

Passive

- [ ] Reading
- [ ] Music
- [ ] TV
- [ ] Light Housework

Date: ____ / ____ / ____   Day ____

Sleep

Bed (last night)	____ am / pm
Asleep	____ am / pm
Woke up	____ am / pm
# of Disruptions	____
Total/Hours slept	____

Medications

☐ No Change in Meds

☐ Dosage Changed

☐ New Medication

Details _____

Today's Ratings

Scale: 0 = None, 10 = Severe

Pain	____ / 10
Fatigue	____ / 10
Weakness	____ / 10
Stiffness	____ / 10
Anxiety	____ / 10
Depression	____ / 10
Stress	____ / 10
Anger	____ / 10
Brain Fog / Forgetfulness	____ / 10

Pain location(s)

Circle or shade in where your pain is using pen, pencil or highlighters

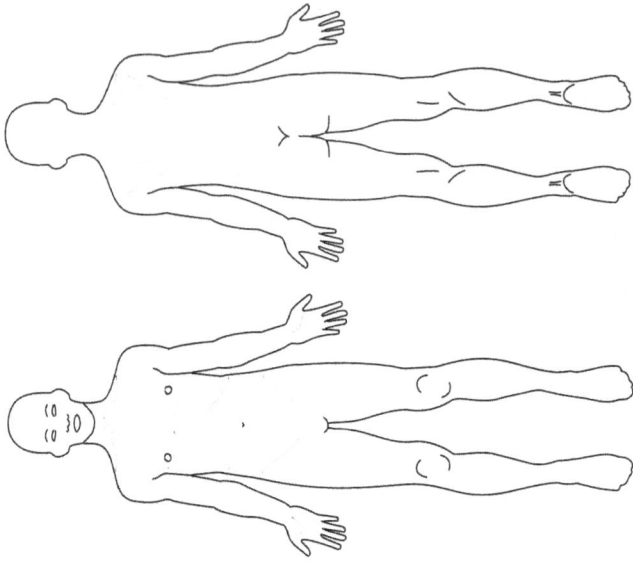

Activity

Active

☐ Walking ☐ Gym
☐ Housework ☐ Hydrotherapy

Passive

☐ Reading ☐ TV
☐ Music ☐ Light Housework

Meals

Breakfast

Lunch

Dinner

Snacks & Dessert

Beverages

☐ Juice ☐ Tea ☐ Water
☐ Milk ☐ Soft D ☐ Coffee
☐ Energy

Symptoms

Date: ___ / ___ / ___   Day ___

Sleep   ## Today's Ratings
                                  Scale: 0 = None, 10 = Severe

Bed (last night) ____ am / pm   Pain ____ / 10

Asleep ____ am / pm   Fatigue ____ / 10

Woke up ____ am / pm   Weakness ____ / 10

# of Disruptions ____   Stiffness ____ / 10

                                  Anxiety ____ / 10

Total/Hours slept ____   Depression ____ / 10

                                  Stress ____ / 10

Medications   Anger ____ / 10

☐ No Change in Meds   Brain Fog / ____ / 10
                                  Forgetfulness
☐ Dosage Changed

☐ New Medication

Details _____

_____

Pain location(s)

Circle or shade in where your pain is using pen, pencil or highlighters

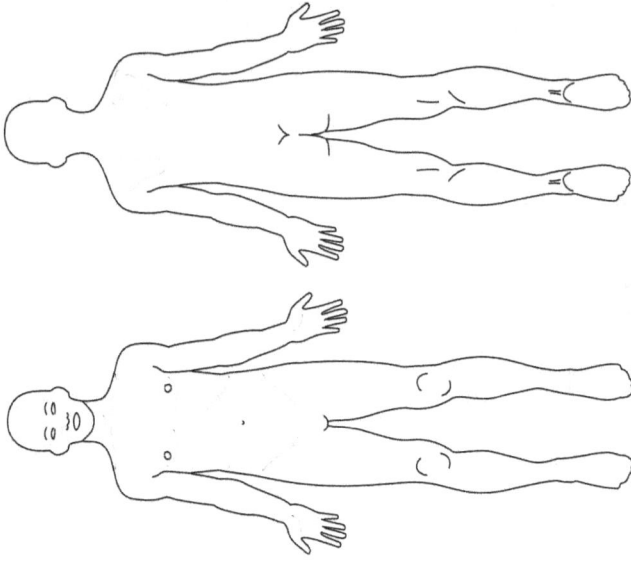

Activity

Active

☐ Walking ☐ Gym
☐ Housework ☐ Hydrotherapy

Passive

☐ Reading ☐ TV
☐ Music ☐ Light Housework

Meals

Breakfast

Lunch

Dinner

Snacks & Dessert

Beverages

☐ Juice ☐ Tea ☐ Water
☐ Milk ☐ Soft D ☐ Coffee
☐ Energy

Symptoms

Date: ____ / ____ / _____ Day ____

Sleep

Bed (last night) _____ am / pm

Asleep _____ am / pm

Woke up _____ am / pm

# of Disruptions _____

Total/Hours slept _____

Medications

☐ No Change in Meds

☐ Dosage Changed

☐ New Medication

Details _____

Today's Ratings

Scale: 0 = None, 10 = Severe

Pain	____ / 10
Fatigue	____ / 10
Weakness	____ / 10
Stiffness	____ / 10
Anxiety	____ / 10
Depression	____ / 10
Stress	____ / 10
Anger	____ / 10
Brain Fog / Forgetfulness	____ / 10

Pain location(s)

Circle or shade in where your pain is using pen, pencil or highlighters

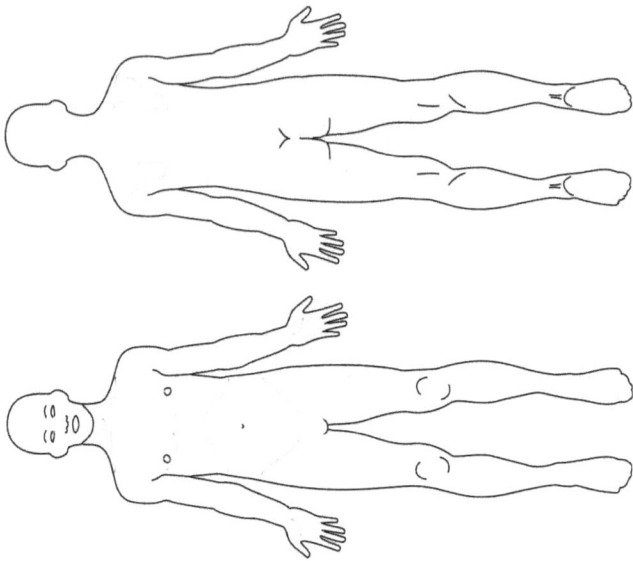

Symptoms

Meals

Breakfast

Lunch

Dinner

Snacks & Dessert

Beverages

☐ Juice ☐ Tea ☐ Water
☐ Milk ☐ Soft D ☐ Coffee
☐ Energy

Activity

Active

☐ Walking ☐ Gym
☐ Housework ☐ Hydrotherapy

Passive

☐ Reading ☐ TV
☐ Music ☐ Light Housework

Date: ___ / ___ / ___

Day ___

Sleep

Bed (last night)	_____ am / pm
Asleep	_____ am / pm
Woke up	_____ am / pm
# of Disruptions	_____
Total Hours slept	_____

Medications

☐ No Change in Meds

☐ Dosage Changed

☐ New Medication

Details _____

Today's Ratings

Scale: 0 = None, 10 = Severe

Pain	___ / 10
Fatigue	___ / 10
Weakness	___ / 10
Stiffness	___ / 10
Anxiety	___ / 10
Depression	___ / 10
Stress	___ / 10
Anger	___ / 10
Brain Fog / Forgetfulness	___ / 10

Pain location(s)

Circle or shade in where your pain is using pen, pencil or highlighters

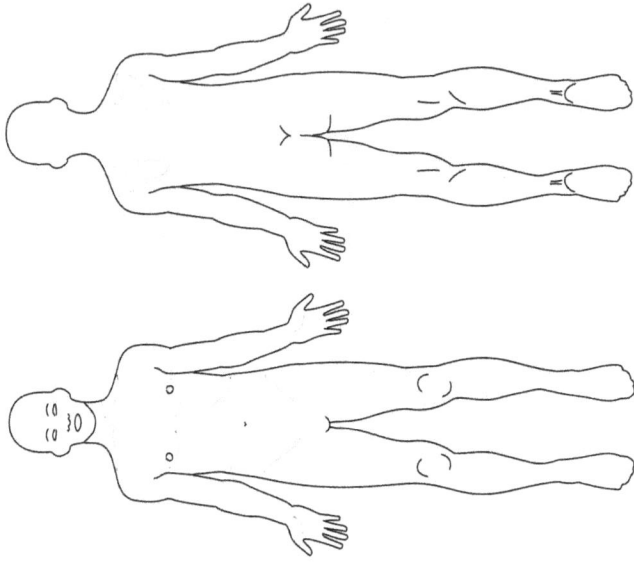

Activity

Active

☐ Walking ☐ Gym
☐ Housework ☐ Hydrotherapy

Passive

☐ Reading ☐ TV
☐ Music ☐ Light Housework

Meals

Breakfast

Lunch

Dinner

Snacks & Dessert

Beverages

☐ Juice ☐ Tea ☐ Water
☐ Milk ☐ Soft D ☐ Coffee
☐ Energy

Symptoms

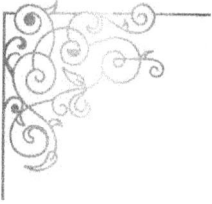

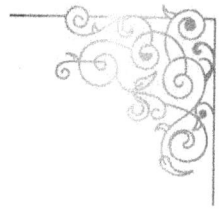

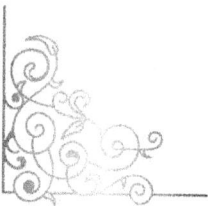

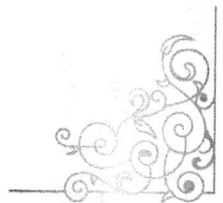

MONTH Two

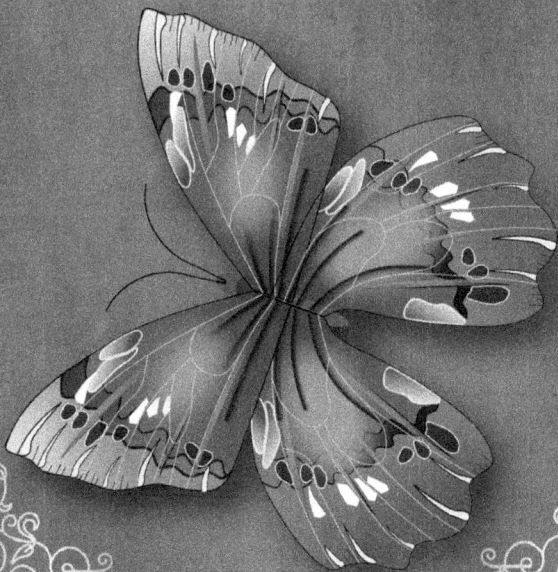

Date: ___ / ___ / ___   Day ___

Sleep

Bed (last night)	___ am / pm
Asleep	___ am / pm
Woke up	___ am / pm
# of Disruptions	___
Total Hours slept	___

Medications

☐ No Change in Meds
☐ Dosage Changed
☐ New Medication

Details _____

Today's Ratings

Scale: 0 = None, 10 = Severe

Pain	___ / 10
Fatigue	___ / 10
Weakness	___ / 10
Stiffness	___ / 10
Anxiety	___ / 10
Depression	___ / 10
Stress	___ / 10
Anger	___ / 10
Brain Fog / Forgetfulness	___ / 10

Pain location(s)

Circle or shade in where your pain is using pen, pencil or highlighters

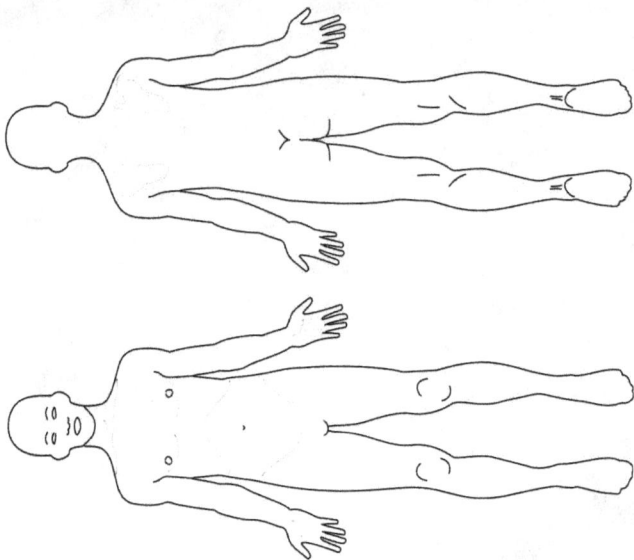

Activity

Active

- [ ] Walking
- [ ] Gym
- [ ] Housework
- [ ] Hydrotherapy

Passive

- [ ] Reading
- [ ] TV
- [ ] Music
- [ ] Light Housework

Meals

Breakfast

Lunch

Dinner

Snacks & Dessert

Beverages

- [ ] Juice
- [ ] Tea
- [ ] Milk
- [ ] Soft D
- [ ] Water
- [ ] Coffee
- [ ] Energy

Symptoms

Date: ___ / ___ / ___

Day ___

Sleep

Bed (last night)	___ am / pm
Asleep	___ am / pm
Woke up	___ am / pm
# of Disruptions	___
Total/Hours slept	___

Medications

☐ No Change in Meds

☐ Dosage Changed

☐ New Medication

Details _____

_____

Today's Ratings

Scale: 0 = None, 10 = Severe

Pain	___ / 10
Fatigue	___ / 10
Weakness	___ / 10
Stiffness	___ / 10
Anxiety	___ / 10
Depression	___ / 10
Stress	___ / 10
Anger	___ / 10
Brain Fog / Forgetfulness	___ / 10

Pain location(s)

Circle or shade in where your pain is using pen, pencil or highlighters

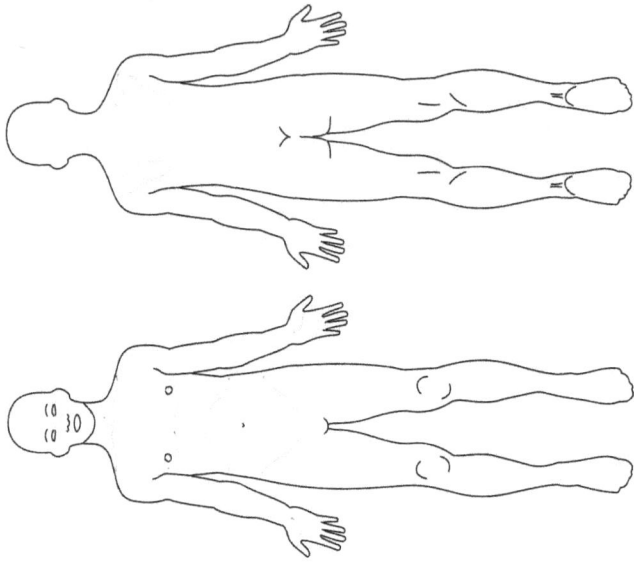

Activity

Active

- [ ] Walking
- [ ] Gym
- [ ] Housework
- [ ] Hydrotherapy

Passive

- [ ] Reading
- [ ] TV
- [ ] Music
- [ ] Light Housework

Meals

Breakfast

Lunch

Dinner

Snacks & Dessert

Beverages

- [ ] Juice
- [ ] Tea
- [ ] Water
- [ ] Milk
- [ ] Soft D
- [ ] Coffee
- [ ] Energy

Symptoms

Date: ___ / ___ / ___

Day ___

Sleep

Bed (last night)	___ am / pm
Asleep	___ am / pm
Woke up	___ am / pm
# of Disruptions	___
Total Hours slept	___

Today's Ratings

Scale: 0 = None, 10 = Severe

Pain	___ /10
Fatigue	___ /10
Weakness	___ /10
Stiffness	___ /10
Anxiety	___ /10
Depression	___ /10
Stress	___ /10
Anger	___ /10
Brain Fog / Forgetfulness	___ /10

Medications

☐ No Change in Meds

☐ Dosage Changed

☐ New Medication

Details

Pain location(s)

Circle or shade in where your pain is using pen, pencil or highlighters

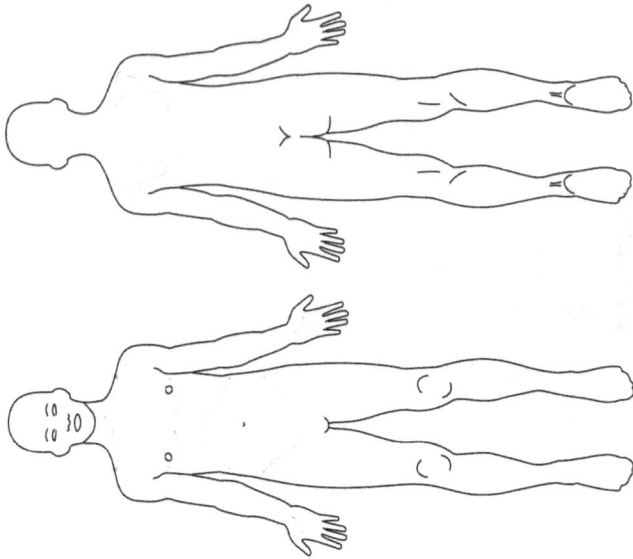

Activity

Active

☐ Walking ☐ Gym

☐ Housework ☐ Hydrotherapy

Passive

☐ Reading ☐ TV

☐ Music ☐ Light Housework

Meals

Breakfast

Lunch

Dinner

Snacks & Dessert

Beverages

☐ Juice ☐ Tea ☐ Water

☐ Milk ☐ Soft D ☐ Coffee

☐ Energy

Symptoms

Date: ___ / ___ / ___   Day ___

Sleep

Bed (last night) _____ am / pm

Asleep _____ am / pm

Woke up _____ am / pm

# of Disruptions _____

Total Hours slept _____

Medications

☐ No Change in Meds

☐ Dosage Changed

☐ New Medication

Details _____

_____

Today's Ratings
Scale: 0 = None, 10 = Severe

Pain _____ / 10

Fatigue _____ / 10

Weakness _____ / 10

Stiffness _____ / 10

Anxiety _____ / 10

Depression _____ / 10

Stress _____ / 10

Anger _____ / 10

Brain Fog / Forgetfulness _____ / 10

Pain location(s)
Circle or shade in where your pain is using pen, pencil or highlighters

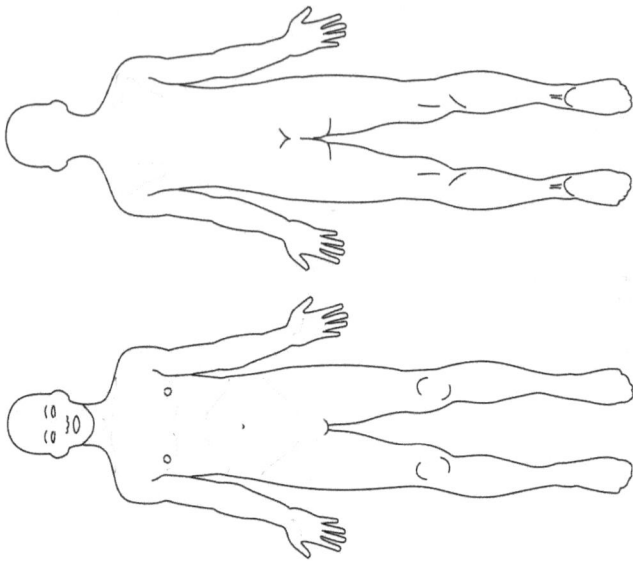

Activity

Active

- [ ] Walking
- [ ] Housework
- [ ] Gym
- [ ] Hydrotherapy

Passive

- [ ] Reading
- [ ] Music
- [ ] TV
- [ ] Light Housework

Meals

Breakfast

Lunch

Dinner

Snacks & Dessert

Beverages

- [ ] Juice
- [ ] Milk
- [ ] Tea
- [ ] Soft D
- [ ] Water
- [ ] Coffee
- [ ] Energy

Symptoms

Date: ____ / ____ / ____   Day ____

Sleep

	am / pm
Bed (last night)	_____
Asleep	_____ am / pm
Woke up	_____ am / pm
# of Disruptions	_____
Total Hours slept	_____

Medications

☐ No Change in Meds

☐ Dosage Changed

☐ New Medication

Details _____

Today's Ratings
Scale: 0 = None, 10 = Severe

Pain	____ / 10
Fatigue	____ / 10
Weakness	____ / 10
Stiffness	____ / 10
Anxiety	____ / 10
Depression	____ / 10
Stress	____ / 10
Anger	____ / 10
Brain Fog / Forgetfulness	____ / 10

Pain location(s)
Circle or shade in where your pain is using pen, pencil or highlighters

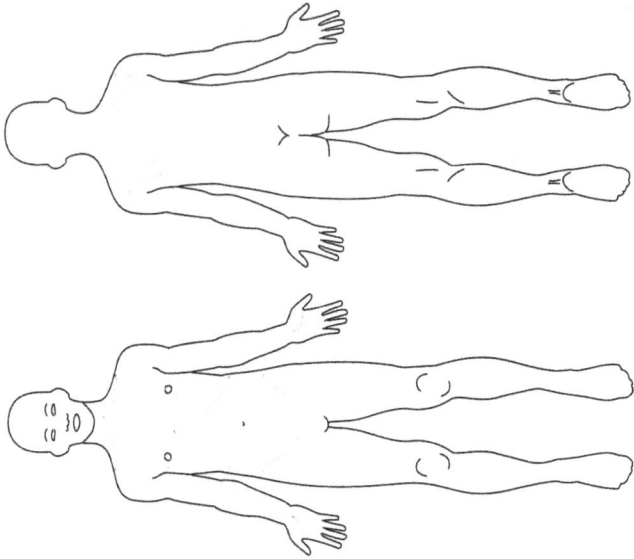

Activity

Active

- [ ] Walking [ ] Gym
- [ ] Housework [ ] Hydrotherapy

Passive

- [ ] Reading [ ] TV
- [ ] Music [ ] Light Housework

Meals

Breakfast

Lunch

Dinner

Snacks & Dessert

Beverages

- [ ] Juice [ ] Tea [ ] Water
- [ ] Milk [ ] Soft D [ ] Coffee
- [ ] Energy

Symptoms

Date: ___ / ___ / ___   Day ____

Sleep

Bed (last night)	_____ am / pm
Asleep	_____ am / pm
Woke up	_____ am / pm
# of Disruptions	_____
Total Hours slept	_____

Medications

☐ No Change in Meds

☐ Dosage Changed

☐ New Medication

Details _____

Today's Ratings

Scale: 0 = None, 10 = Severe

Pain	___ / 10
Fatigue	___ / 10
Weakness	___ / 10
Stiffness	___ / 10
Anxiety	___ / 10
Depression	___ / 10
Stress	___ / 10
Anger	___ / 10
Brain Fog / Forgetfulness	___ / 10

Pain location(s)

Circle or shade in where your pain is using pen, pencil or highlighters

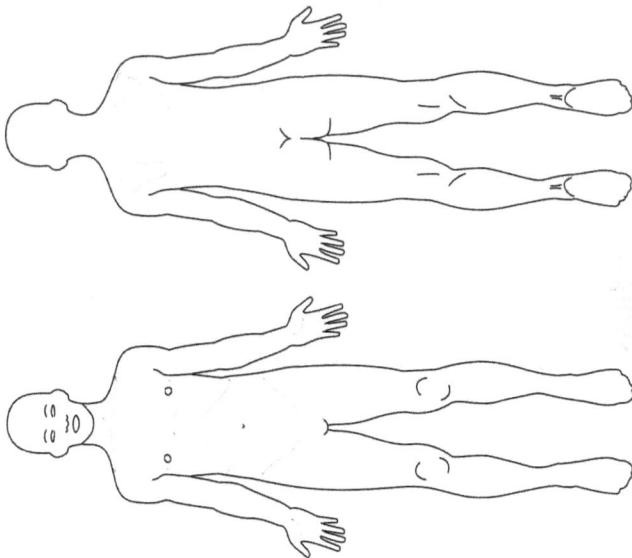

Activity

Active

- [ ] Walking
- [ ] Gym
- [ ] Housework
- [ ] Hydrotherapy

Passive

- [ ] Reading
- [ ] TV
- [ ] Music
- [ ] Light Housework

Meals

Breakfast

Lunch

Dinner

Snacks & Dessert

Beverages

- [ ] Juice
- [ ] Tea
- [ ] Water
- [ ] Milk
- [ ] Soft D
- [ ] Coffee
- [ ] Energy

Symptoms

Date: ___ / ___ / ___

Day ___

Sleep

Bed (last night)	_____ am / pm
Asleep	_____ am / pm
Woke up	_____ am / pm
# of Disruptions	_____
Total/Hours slept	_____

Medications

☐ No Change in Meds

☐ Dosage Changed

☐ New Medication

Details _____

Today's Ratings

Scale: 0 = None, 10 = Severe

Pain	_____ / 10
Fatigue	_____ / 10
Weakness	_____ / 10
Stiffness	_____ / 10
Anxiety	_____ / 10
Depression	_____ / 10
Stress	_____ / 10
Anger	_____ / 10
Brain Fog / Forgetfulness	_____ / 10

Pain location(s)

Circle or shade in where your pain is using pen, pencil or highlighters

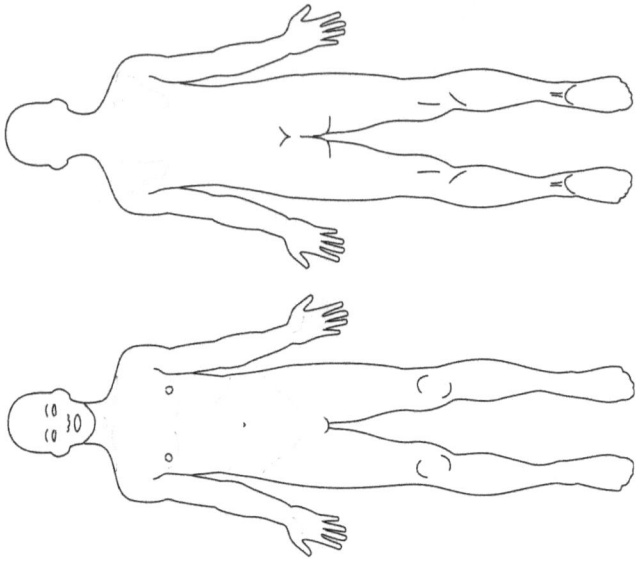

Symptoms

Meals

Breakfast

Lunch

Dinner

Snacks & Dessert

Beverages

☐ Juice   ☐ Tea   ☐ Water

☐ Milk   ☐ Soft D   ☐ Coffee

☐ Energy

Activity

Active

☐ Walking   ☐ Gym

☐ Housework   ☐ Hydrotherapy

Passive

☐ Reading   ☐ TV

☐ Music   ☐ Light Housework

Date: ___ / ___ / ___   Day ___

Sleep

Bed (last night)	_____ am / pm
Asleep	_____ am / pm
Woke up	_____ am / pm
# of Disruptions	_____
Total/Hours slept	_____

Medications

☐ No Change in Meds
☐ Dosage Changed
☐ New Medication

Details _____
_____

Today's Ratings

Scale: 0 = None, 10 = Severe

Pain	___ / 10
Fatigue	___ / 10
Weakness	___ / 10
Stiffness	___ / 10
Anxiety	___ / 10
Depression	___ / 10
Stress	___ / 10
Anger	___ / 10
Brain Fog / Forgetfulness	___ / 10

Pain location(s)

Circle or shade in where your pain is using pen, pencil or highlighters

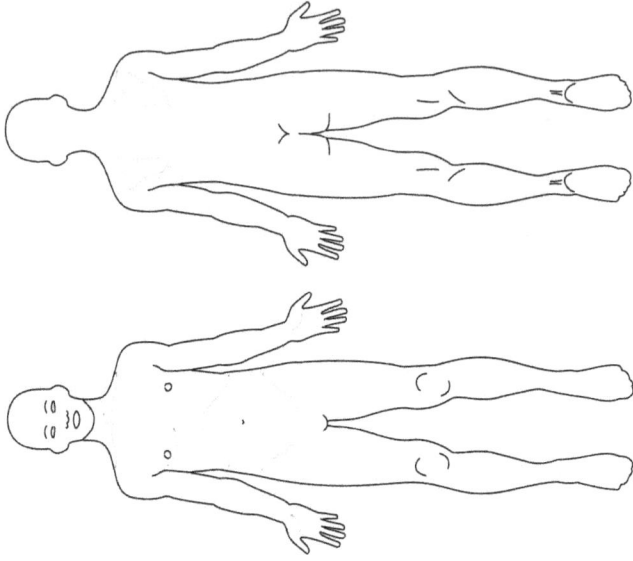

Activity

Active

☐ Walking ☐ Gym
☐ Housework ☐ Hydrotherapy

Passive

☐ Reading ☐ TV
☐ Music ☐ Light Housework

Meals

Breakfast

Lunch

Dinner

Snacks & Dessert

Beverages

☐ Juice ☐ Tea ☐ Water
☐ Milk ☐ Soft D ☐ Coffee
☐ Energy

Symptoms

Date: ___ / ___ / ___

Day ___

Sleep

Bed (last night)	___ am / pm
Asleep	___ am / pm
Woke up	___ am / pm
# of Disruptions	___
Total Hours slept	___

Medications

☐ No Change in Meds

☐ Dosage Changed

☐ New Medication

Details

_____

_____

Today's Ratings

Scale: 0 = None, 10 = Severe

Pain	___ / 10
Fatigue	___ / 10
Weakness	___ / 10
Stiffness	___ / 10
Anxiety	___ / 10
Depression	___ / 10
Stress	___ / 10
Anger	___ / 10
Brain Fog / Forgetfulness	___ / 10

Pain location(s)

Circle or shade in where your pain is using pen, pencil or highlighters

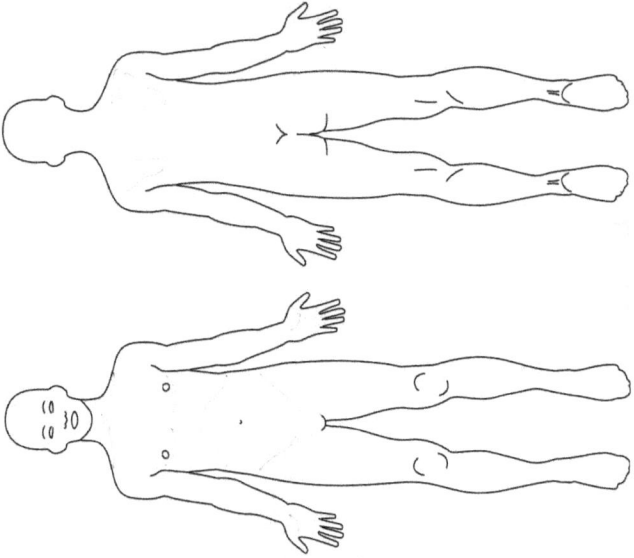

Symptoms

Meals

Breakfast

Lunch

Dinner

Snacks & Dessert

Beverages

- [ ] Juice
- [ ] Milk
- [ ] Tea
- [ ] Soft D
- [ ] Water
- [ ] Coffee
- [ ] Energy

Activity

Active

- [ ] Walking
- [ ] Housework
- [ ] Gym
- [ ] Hydrotherapy

Passive

- [ ] Reading
- [ ] Music
- [ ] TV
- [ ] Light Housework

Date: ___ / ___ / ___   Day ___

Sleep

Bed (last night)	___ am / pm
Asleep	___ am / pm
Woke up	___ am / pm
# of Disruptions	___
Total Hours slept	___

Medications

☐ No Change in Meds

☐ Dosage Changed

☐ New Medication

Details _____

Today's Ratings

Scale: 0 = None, 10 = Severe

Pain	___ / 10
Fatigue	___ / 10
Weakness	___ / 10
Stiffness	___ / 10
Anxiety	___ / 10
Depression	___ / 10
Stress	___ / 10
Anger	___ / 10
Brain Fog / Forgetfulness	___ / 10

Pain location(s)

Circle or shade in where your pain is using pen, pencil or highlighters

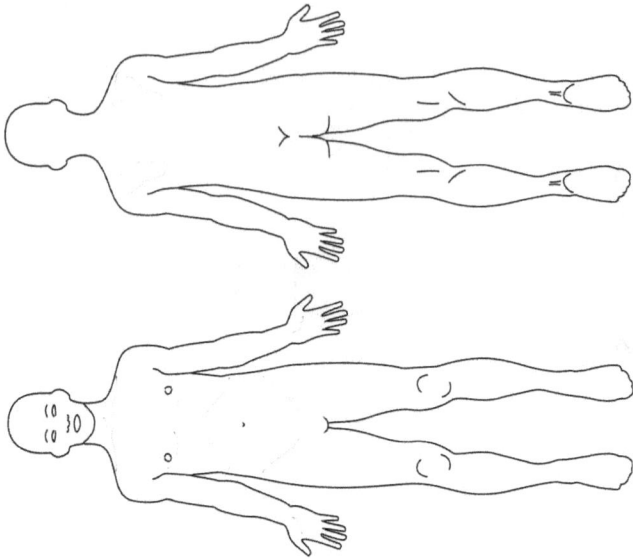

Activity

Active

☐ Walking ☐ Gym
☐ Housework ☐ Hydrotherapy

Passive

☐ Reading ☐ TV
☐ Music ☐ Light Housework

Meals

Breakfast

Lunch

Dinner

Snacks & Dessert

Beverages

☐ Juice ☐ Tea ☐ Water
☐ Milk ☐ Soft D ☐ Coffee
☐ Energy

Symptoms

Date: ___ / ___ / ___

Day ____

Sleep

Bed (last night)	___ am / pm
Asleep	___ am / pm
Woke up	___ am / pm
# of Disruptions	___
Total/Hours slept	___

Medications

☐ No Change in Meds

☐ Dosage Changed

☐ New Medication

Details _____

Today's Ratings
Scale: 0 = None, 10 = Severe

Pain	___ / 10
Fatigue	___ / 10
Weakness	___ / 10
Stiffness	___ / 10
Anxiety	___ / 10
Depression	___ / 10
Stress	___ / 10
Anger	___ / 10
Brain Fog / Forgetfulness	___ / 10

Pain location(s)
Circle or shade in where your pain is using pen, pencil or highlighters

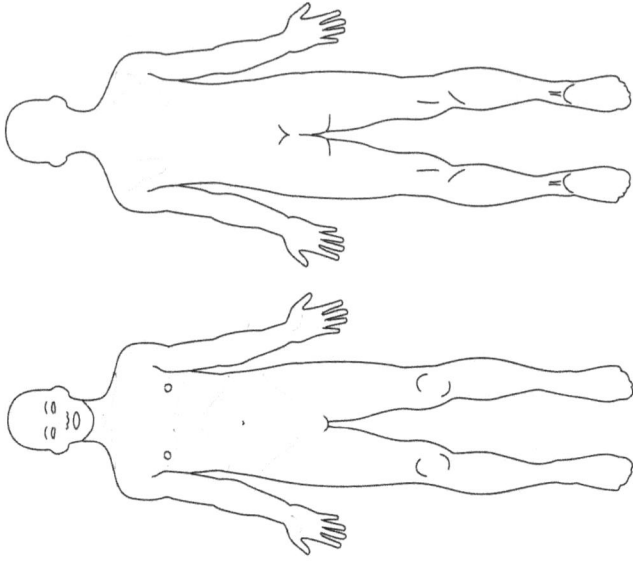

Symptoms

Meals

Breakfast

Lunch

Dinner

Snacks & Dessert

Beverages

- [ ] Juice
- [ ] Milk
- [ ] Tea
- [ ] Soft D
- [ ] Water
- [ ] Coffee
- [ ] Energy

Activity

Active

- [ ] Walking
- [ ] Housework
- [ ] Gym
- [ ] Hydrotherapy

Passive

- [ ] Reading
- [ ] Music
- [ ] TV
- [ ] Light Housework

Date: ___ / ___ / ___

Day ___

Sleep

Bed (last night)	___ am / pm
Asleep	___ am / pm
Woke up	___ am / pm
# of Disruptions	___
Total/Hours slept	___

Medications

☐ No Change in Meds

☐ Dosage Changed

☐ New Medication

Details

_____

_____

Today's Ratings

Scale: 0 = None, 10 = Severe

Pain	___ / 10
Fatigue	___ / 10
Weakness	___ / 10
Stiffness	___ / 10
Anxiety	___ / 10
Depression	___ / 10
Stress	___ / 10
Anger	___ / 10
Brain Fog / Forgetfulness	___ / 10

Pain location(s)

Circle or shade in where your pain is using pen, pencil or highlighters

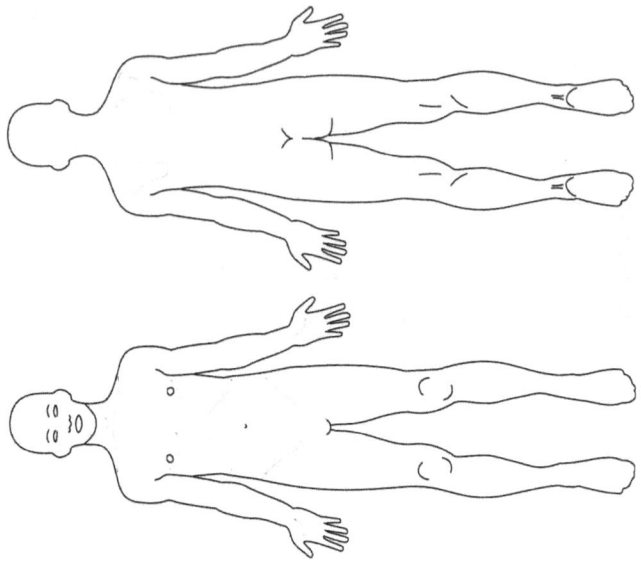

Symptoms

Meals

Breakfast

Lunch

Dinner

Snacks & Dessert

Beverages

- [ ] Juice
- [ ] Milk
- [ ] Tea
- [ ] Soft D
- [ ] Water
- [ ] Coffee
- [ ] Energy

Activity

Active

- [ ] Walking
- [ ] Housework
- [ ] Gym
- [ ] Hydrotherapy

Passive

- [ ] Reading
- [ ] Music
- [ ] TV
- [ ] Light Housework

Date: _____ / _____ / _____

Day _____

Sleep

Bed (last night) _____ am / pm

Asleep _____ am / pm

Woke up _____ am / pm

# of Disruptions _____

Total Hours slept _____

Medications

☐ No Change in Meds

☐ Dosage Changed

☐ New Medication

Details _____

_____

Today's Ratings

Scale: 0 = None, 10 = Severe

Pain _____ / 10

Fatigue _____ / 10

Weakness _____ / 10

Stiffness _____ / 10

Anxiety _____ / 10

Depression _____ / 10

Stress _____ / 10

Anger _____ / 10

Brain Fog / Forgetfulness _____ / 10

Pain location(s)

Circle or shade in where your pain is using pen, pencil or highlighters

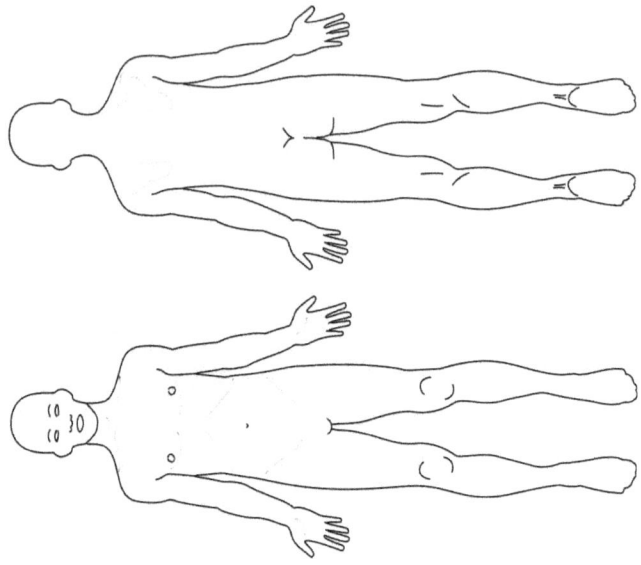

Symptoms

Meals

Breakfast

Lunch

Dinner

Snacks & Dessert

Beverages

- [ ] Juice
- [ ] Tea
- [ ] Water
- [ ] Milk
- [ ] Soft D
- [ ] Coffee
- [ ] Energy

Activity

Active

- [ ] Walking
- [ ] Gym
- [ ] Housework
- [ ] Hydrotherapy

Passive

- [ ] Reading
- [ ] TV
- [ ] Music
- [ ] Light Housework

Date: ___ / ___ / ___

Day ___

Sleep

Bed (last night)	_____ am / pm
Asleep	_____ am / pm
Woke up	_____ am / pm
# of Disruptions	_____
Total Hours slept	_____

Today's Ratings
Scale: 0 = None, 10 = Severe

Pain	_____ / 10
Fatigue	_____ / 10
Weakness	_____ / 10
Stiffness	_____ / 10
Anxiety	_____ / 10
Depression	_____ / 10
Stress	_____ / 10
Anger	_____ / 10
Brain Fog / Forgetfulness	_____ / 10

Medications

☐ No Change in Meds

☐ Dosage Changed

☐ New Medication

Details

_____

Pain location(s)
Circle or shade in where your pain is using pen, pencil or highlighters

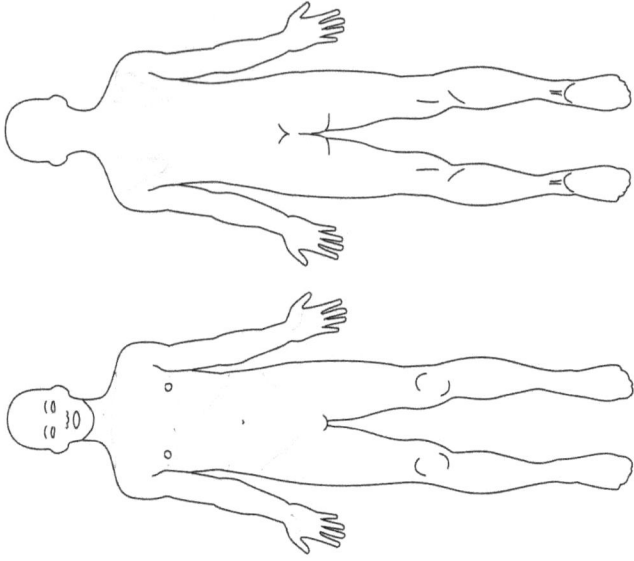

Symptoms

Meals

Breakfast

Lunch

Dinner

Snacks & Dessert

Beverages

- [ ] Juice
- [ ] Tea
- [ ] Water
- [ ] Milk
- [ ] Soft D
- [ ] Coffee
- [ ] Energy

Activity

Active

- [ ] Walking
- [ ] Gym
- [ ] Housework
- [ ] Hydrotherapy

Passive

- [ ] Reading
- [ ] TV
- [ ] Music
- [ ] Light Housework

Date: ___ / ___ / ___   Day ___

Sleep

Bed (last night)	_____ am / pm
Asleep	_____ am / pm
Woke up	_____ am / pm
# of Disruptions	_____
Total/Hours slept	_____

Today's Ratings
Scale: 0 = None, 10 = Severe

Pain	____ / 10
Fatigue	____ / 10
Weakness	____ / 10
Stiffness	____ / 10
Anxiety	____ / 10
Depression	____ / 10
Stress	____ / 10
Anger	____ / 10
Brain Fog /	____ / 10
Forgetfulness	

Medications

☐ No Change in Meds

☐ Dosage Changed

☐ New Medication

Details _____

_____

Pain location(s)

Circle or shade in where your pain is using pen, pencil or highlighters

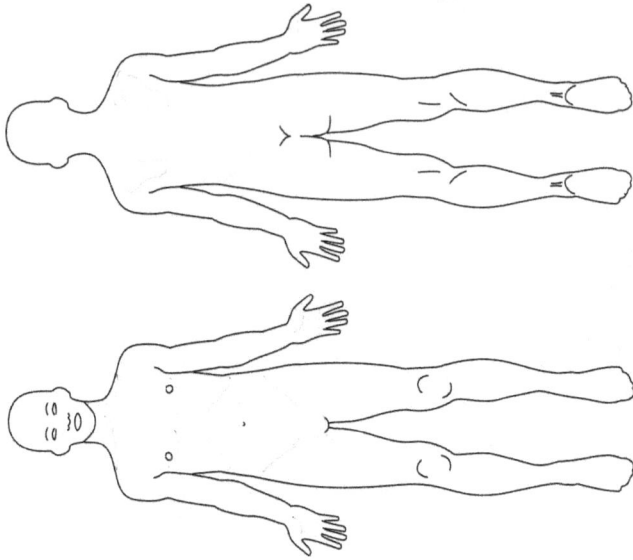

Activity

Active
- ☐ Walking ☐ Gym
- ☐ Housework ☐ Hydrotherapy

Passive
- ☐ Reading ☐ TV
- ☐ Music ☐ Light Housework

Meals

Breakfast

Lunch

Dinner

Snacks & Dessert

Beverages
- ☐ Juice ☐ Tea ☐ Water
- ☐ Milk ☐ Soft D ☐ Coffee
- ☐ Energy

Symptoms

Date: ___ / ___ / ___

Day ___

Sleep

Bed (last night)	___ am / pm
Asleep	___ am / pm
Woke up	___ am / pm
# of Disruptions	___
Total Hours slept	___

Today's Ratings

Scale: 0 = None, 10 = Severe

Pain	___ / 10
Fatigue	___ / 10
Weakness	___ / 10
Stiffness	___ / 10
Anxiety	___ / 10
Depression	___ / 10
Stress	___ / 10
Anger	___ / 10
Brain Fog / Forgetfulness	___ / 10

Medications

☐ No Change in Meds

☐ Dosage Changed

☐ New Medication

Details

Pain location(s)

Circle or shade in where your pain is using pen, pencil or highlighters

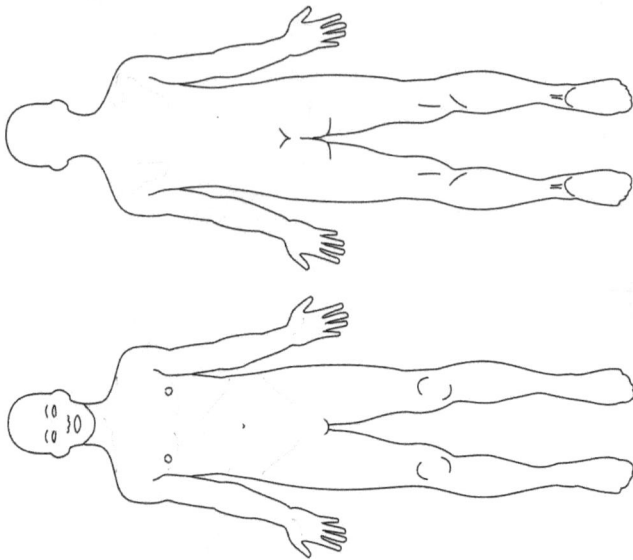

Symptoms

Meals

Breakfast

Lunch

Dinner

Snacks & Dessert

Beverages

☐ Juice ☐ Tea ☐ Water

☐ Milk ☐ Soft D ☐ Coffee

☐ Energy

Activity

Active

☐ Walking ☐ Gym

☐ Housework ☐ Hydrotherapy

Passive

☐ Reading ☐ TV

☐ Music ☐ Light Housework

Date: ___ / ___ / ___

Sleep

Bed (last night) _____ am / pm

Asleep _____ am / pm

Woke up _____ am / pm

# of Disruptions _____

Total/Hours slept _____

Medications

☐ No Change in Meds

☐ Dosage Changed

☐ New Medication

Details _____

_____

Today's Ratings

Scale: 0 = None, 10 = Severe

Pain	___ / 10
Fatigue	___ / 10
Weakness	___ / 10
Stiffness	___ / 10
Anxiety	___ / 10
Depression	___ / 10
Stress	___ / 10
Anger	___ / 10
Brain Fog / Forgetfulness	___ / 10

Pain location(s)

Circle or shade in where your pain is using pen, pencil or highlighters

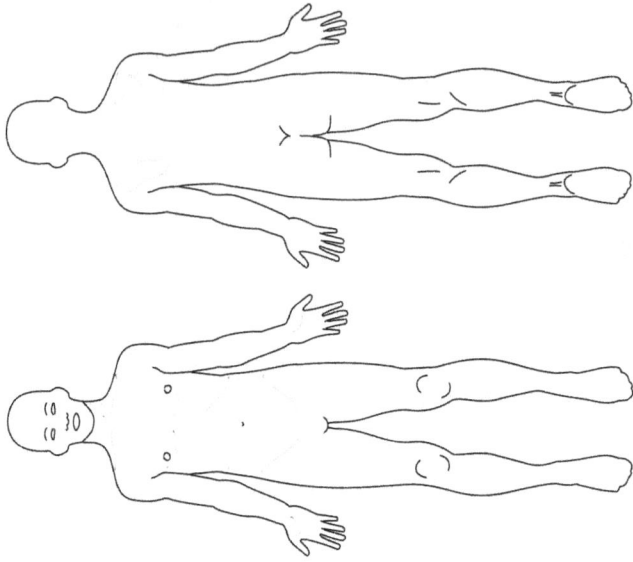

Day ____

Symptoms

Meals

Breakfast

Lunch

Dinner

Snacks & Dessert

Beverages

- [ ] Juice
- [ ] Milk
- [ ] Tea
- [ ] Soft D
- [ ] Water
- [ ] Coffee
- [ ] Energy

Activity

Active

- [ ] Walking
- [ ] Housework
- [ ] Gym
- [ ] Hydrotherapy

Passive

- [ ] Reading
- [ ] Music
- [ ] TV
- [ ] Light Housework

Date: ___ / ___ / ___   Day ___

Sleep

Bed (last night) _____ am / pm

Asleep _____ am / pm

Woke up _____ am / pm

# of Disruptions _____

Total/Hours slept _____

Medications

☐ No Change in Meds

☐ Dosage Changed

☐ New Medication

Details

_____

_____

Today's Ratings

Scale: 0 = None, 10 = Severe

Pain _____ / 10

Fatigue _____ / 10

Weakness _____ / 10

Stiffness _____ / 10

Anxiety _____ / 10

Depression _____ / 10

Stress _____ / 10

Anger _____ / 10

Brain Fog / _____ / 10
Forgetfulness

Pain location(s)

Circle or shade in where your pain is using pen, pencil or highlighters

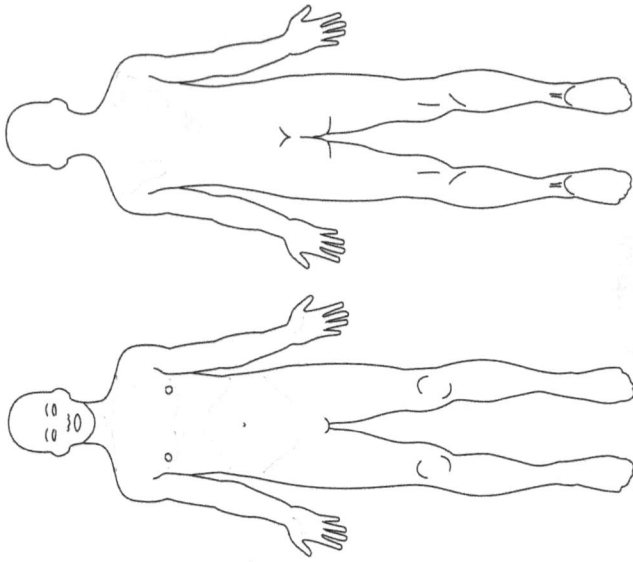

Symptoms

Meals

Breakfast

Lunch

Dinner

Snacks & Dessert

Beverages

☐ Juice ☐ Tea ☐ Water
☐ Milk ☐ Soft D ☐ Coffee
☐ Energy

Activity

Active

☐ Walking ☐ Gym
☐ Housework ☐ Hydrotherapy

Passive

☐ Reading ☐ TV
☐ Music ☐ Light Housework

Date: ___ / ___ / ___

Day ___

Sleep

Bed (last night)	___ am / pm
Asleep	___ am / pm
Woke up	___ am / pm
# of Disruptions	___
Total Hours slept	___

Today's Ratings

Scale: 0 = None, 10 = Severe

Pain	___ / 10
Fatigue	___ / 10
Weakness	___ / 10
Stiffness	___ / 10
Anxiety	___ / 10
Depression	___ / 10
Stress	___ / 10
Anger	___ / 10
Brain Fog / Forgetfulness	___ / 10

Medications

☐ No Change in Meds

☐ Dosage Changed

☐ New Medication

Details

Pain location(s)

Circle or shade in where your pain is using pen, pencil or highlighters

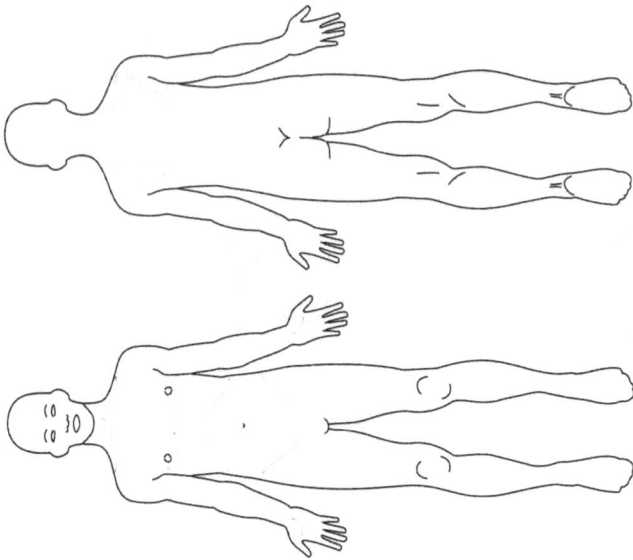

Symptoms

Meals

Breakfast

Lunch

Dinner

Snacks & Dessert

Beverages

- [ ] Juice
- [ ] Milk
- [ ] Tea
- [ ] Soft D
- [ ] Water
- [ ] Coffee
- [ ] Energy

Activity

Active

- [ ] Walking
- [ ] Housework
- [ ] Gym
- [ ] Hydrotherapy

Passive

- [ ] Reading
- [ ] Music
- [ ] TV
- [ ] Light Housework

Date: ___ / ___ / ___   Day ___

Sleep

Bed (last night)	_____ am / pm
Asleep	_____ am / pm
Woke up	_____ am / pm
# of Disruptions	_____
Total Hours slept	_____

Medications

☐ No Change in Meds

☐ Dosage Changed

☐ New Medication

Details _____

_____

Today's Ratings

Scale: 0 = None, 10 = Severe

Pain	___ / 10
Fatigue	___ / 10
Weakness	___ / 10
Stiffness	___ / 10
Anxiety	___ / 10
Depression	___ / 10
Stress	___ / 10
Anger	___ / 10
Brain Fog / Forgetfulness	___ / 10

Pain location(s)

Circle or shade in where your pain is using pen, pencil or highlighters

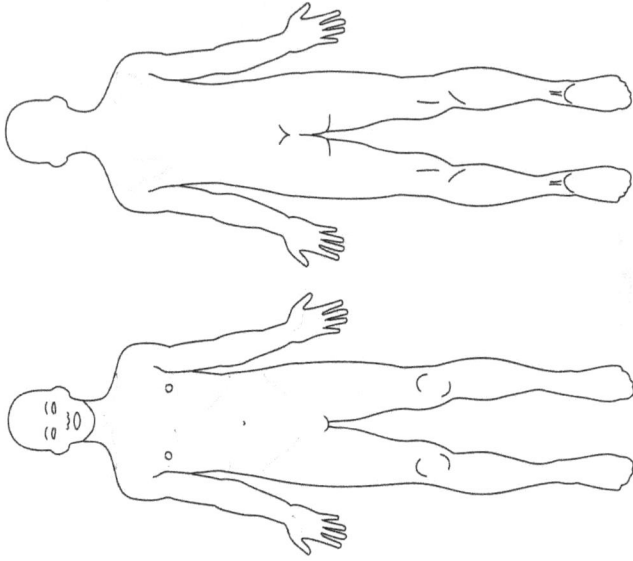

Symptoms

_____
_____
_____
_____
_____
_____
_____
_____
_____
_____

Meals

Breakfast
_____

Lunch
_____

Dinner
_____

Snacks & Dessert
_____

Beverages

☐ Juice   ☐ Tea   ☐ Water
☐ Milk   ☐ Soft D ☐ Coffee
                     ☐ Energy

Activity

Active

☐ Walking   ☐ Gym
☐ Housework ☐ Hydrotherapy

_____
_____

Passive

☐ Reading ☐ TV
☐ Music   ☐ Light Housework

_____
_____

Date: ___ / ___ / ___   Day ____

Sleep   ## Today's Ratings
                            Scale: 0 = None, 10 = Severe

Bed (last night) _____ am / pm   Pain _____ / 10

Asleep _____ am / pm   Fatigue _____ / 10

Woke up _____ am / pm   Weakness _____ / 10

# of Disruptions _____   Stiffness _____ / 10

                                  Anxiety _____ / 10

Total Hours slept _____   Depression _____ / 10

                                  Stress _____ / 10

Medications   Anger _____ / 10

☐ No Change in Meds   Brain Fog / _____ / 10
                                  Forgetfulness
☐ Dosage Changed

☐ New Medication

Details

Pain location(s)

Circle or shade in where your pain is using pen, pencil or highlighters

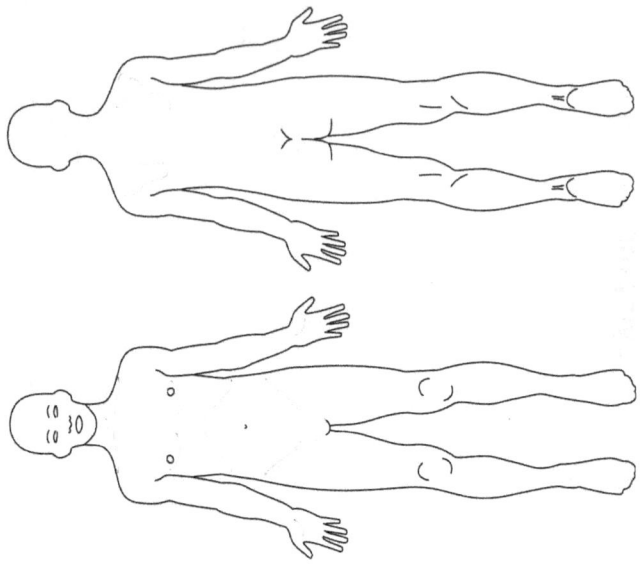

Activity

Active

- [ ] Walking
- [ ] Gym
- [ ] Housework
- [ ] Hydrotherapy

Passive

- [ ] Reading
- [ ] TV
- [ ] Music
- [ ] Light Housework

Meals

Breakfast

Lunch

Dinner

Snacks & Dessert

Beverages

- [ ] Juice
- [ ] Tea
- [ ] Milk
- [ ] Soft D
- [ ] Water
- [ ] Coffee
- [ ] Energy

Symptoms

Date: ___ / ___ / ___

Day ___

Sleep

Bed (last night)	___ am / pm
Asleep	___ am / pm
Woke up	___ am / pm
# of Disruptions	___
Total Hours slept	___

Medications

☐ No Change in Meds

☐ Dosage Changed

☐ New Medication

Details

Today's Ratings

Scale: 0 = None, 10 = Severe

Pain	___ / 10
Fatigue	___ / 10
Weakness	___ / 10
Stiffness	___ / 10
Anxiety	___ / 10
Depression	___ / 10
Stress	___ / 10
Anger	___ / 10
Brain Fog / Forgetfulness	___ / 10

Pain location(s)

Circle or shade in where your pain is using pen, pencil or highlighters

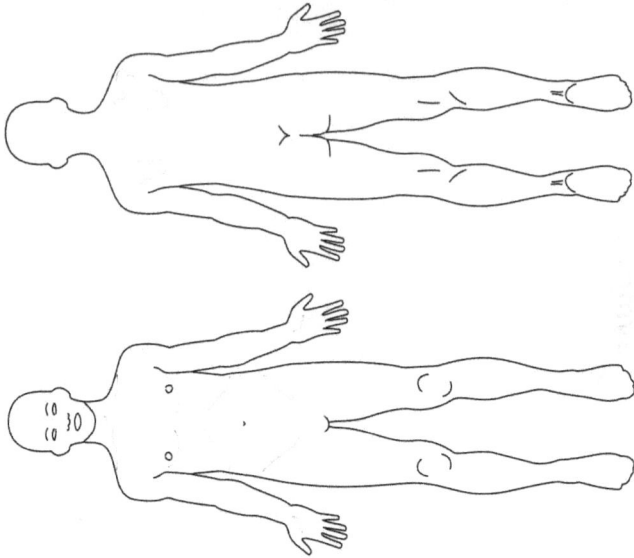

Activity

Active

☐ Walking ☐ Gym
☐ Housework ☐ Hydrotherapy

Passive

☐ Reading ☐ TV
☐ Music ☐ Light Housework

Meals

Breakfast

Lunch

Dinner

Snacks & Dessert

Beverages

☐ Juice ☐ Tea ☐ Water
☐ Milk ☐ Soft D ☐ Coffee
☐ Energy

Symptoms

Date: ___ / ___ / ___   Day ___

Sleep

Bed (last night) _____ am / pm

Asleep _____ am / pm

Woke up _____ am / pm

# of Disruptions _____

Total Hours slept _____

Medications

☐ No Change in Meds

☐ Dosage Changed

☐ New Medication

Details _____

Today's Ratings

Scale: 0 = None, 10 = Severe

Pain _____ / 10

Fatigue _____ / 10

Weakness _____ / 10

Stiffness _____ / 10

Anxiety _____ / 10

Depression _____ / 10

Stress _____ / 10

Anger _____ / 10

Brain Fog / Forgetfulness _____ / 10

Pain location(s)

Circle or shade in where your pain is using pen, pencil or highlighters

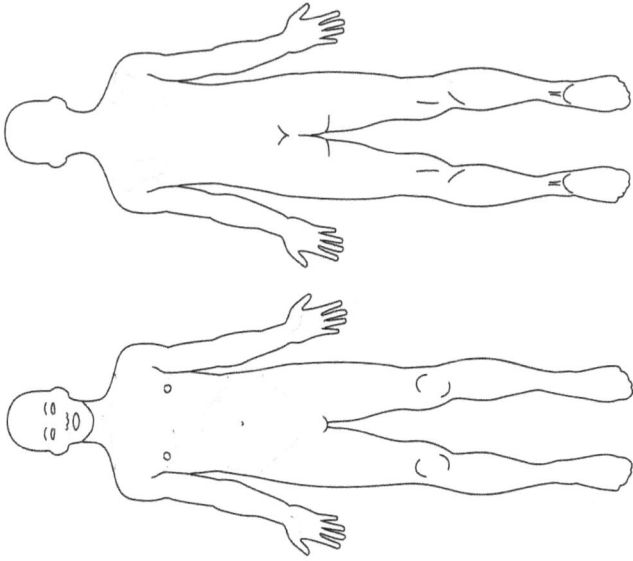

Activity

Active

- [ ] Walking
- [ ] Housework
- [ ] Gym
- [ ] Hydrotherapy

Passive

- [ ] Reading
- [ ] Music
- [ ] TV
- [ ] Light Housework

Meals

Breakfast

Lunch

Dinner

Snacks & Dessert

Beverages

- [ ] Juice
- [ ] Milk
- [ ] Tea
- [ ] Soft D
- [ ] Water
- [ ] Coffee
- [ ] Energy

Symptoms

Date: ___ / ___ / ___   Day ___

Sleep

Bed (last night)	___ am / pm
Asleep	___ am / pm
Woke up	___ am / pm
# of Disruptions	___
Total Hours slept	___

Medications

☐ No Change in Meds

☐ Dosage Changed

☐ New Medication

Details _____

_____

Today's Ratings

Scale: 0 = None, 10 = Severe

Pain	___ / 10
Fatigue	___ / 10
Weakness	___ / 10
Stiffness	___ / 10
Anxiety	___ / 10
Depression	___ / 10
Stress	___ / 10
Anger	___ / 10
Brain Fog / Forgetfulness	___ / 10

Pain location(s)

Circle or shade in where your pain is using pen, pencil or highlighters

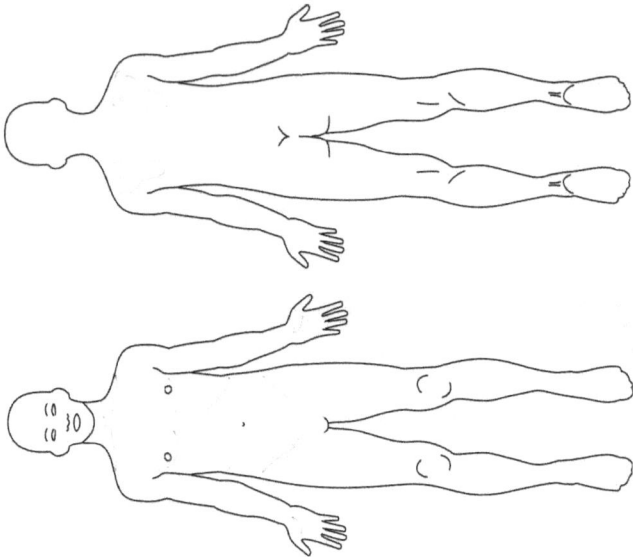

Activity

Active

- [ ] Walking [ ] Gym
- [ ] Housework [ ] Hydrotherapy

Passive

- [ ] Reading [ ] TV
- [ ] Music [ ] Light Housework

Meals

Breakfast

Lunch

Dinner

Snacks & Dessert

Beverages

- [ ] Juice [ ] Tea [ ] Water
- [ ] Milk [ ] Soft D [ ] Coffee
- [ ] Energy

Symptoms

Date: _____ / _____ / _____   Day _____

Sleep

Bed (last night) _____ am / pm

Asleep _____ am / pm

Woke up _____ am / pm

# of Disruptions _____

Total/Hours slept _____

Medications

☐ No Change in Meds

☐ Dosage Changed

☐ New Medication

Details

Today's Ratings

Scale: 0 = None, 10 = Severe

Pain _____ / 10

Fatigue _____ / 10

Weakness _____ / 10

Stiffness _____ / 10

Anxiety _____ / 10

Depression _____ / 10

Stress _____ / 10

Anger _____ / 10

Brain Fog / _____ / 10
Forgetfulness

Pain location(s)

Circle or shade in where your pain is using pen, pencil or highlighters

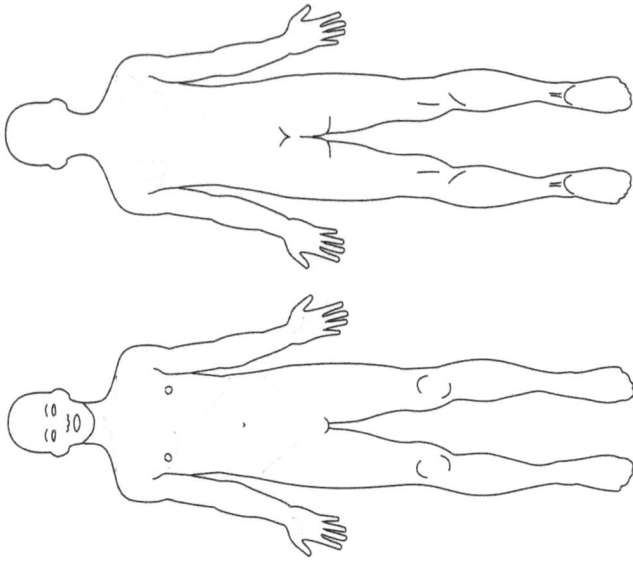

Meals

Symptoms

Breakfast

Lunch

Dinner

Snacks & Dessert

Beverages

☐ Juice ☐ Tea ☐ Water

☐ Milk ☐ Soft D ☐ Coffee

☐ Energy

Activity

Active

☐ Walking ☐ Gym

☐ Housework ☐ Hydrotherapy

Passive

☐ Reading ☐ TV

☐ Music ☐ Light Housework

Date: ___ / ___ / ___   Day ___

Sleep

Bed (last night) _____ am / pm

Asleep _____ am / pm

Woke up _____ am / pm

# of Disruptions _____

Total Hours slept _____

Medications

☐ No Change in Meds

☐ Dosage Changed

☐ New Medication

Details _____

_____

Today's Ratings
Scale: 0 = None, 10 = Severe

Pain _____ / 10

Fatigue _____ / 10

Weakness _____ / 10

Stiffness _____ / 10

Anxiety _____ / 10

Depression _____ / 10

Stress _____ / 10

Anger _____ / 10

Brain Fog / _____ / 10
Forgetfulness

Pain location(s)

Circle or shade in where your pain is using pen, pencil or highlighters

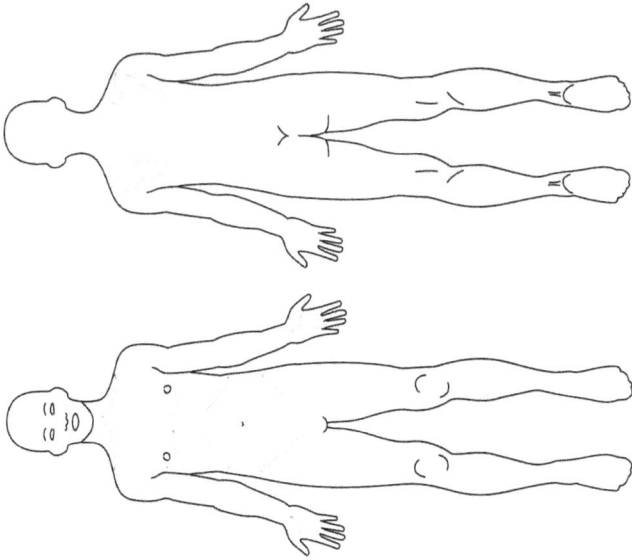

Symptoms

Meals

Breakfast

Lunch

Dinner

Snacks & Dessert

Beverages

☐ Juice ☐ Tea ☐ Water
☐ Milk ☐ Soft D ☐ Coffee
☐ Energy

Activity

Active

☐ Walking ☐ Gym
☐ Housework ☐ Hydrotherapy

Passive

☐ Reading ☐ TV
☐ Music ☐ Light Housework

Date: ___ / ___ / ___

Day ___

Sleep

Bed (last night)	_____ am / pm
Asleep	_____ am / pm
Woke up	_____ am / pm
# of Disruptions	_____
Total/Hours slept	_____

Today's Ratings
Scale: 0 = None, 10 = Severe

Pain	_____ / 10
Fatigue	_____ / 10
Weakness	_____ / 10
Stiffness	_____ / 10
Anxiety	_____ / 10
Depression	_____ / 10
Stress	_____ / 10
Anger	_____ / 10
Brain Fog / Forgetfulness	_____ / 10

Medications

☐ No Change in Meds

☐ Dosage Changed

☐ New Medication

Details _____

_____

Pain location(s)
Circle or shade in where your pain is using pen, pencil or highlighters

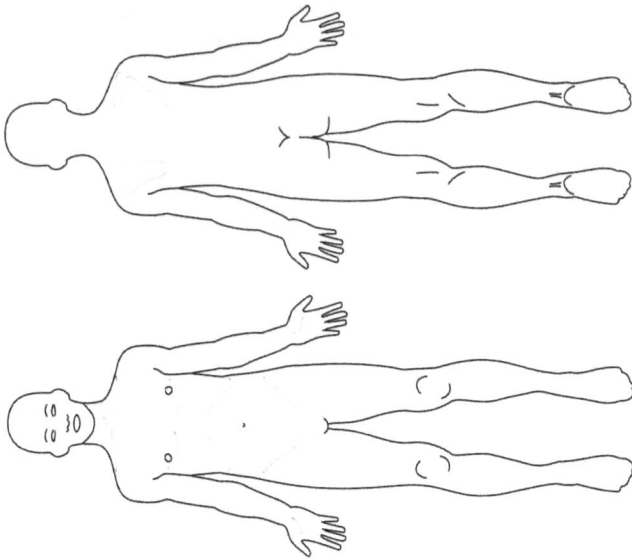

Activity

Active

- [ ] Walking
- [ ] Gym
- [ ] Housework
- [ ] Hydrotherapy

Passive

- [ ] Reading
- [ ] TV
- [ ] Music
- [ ] Light Housework

Meals

Breakfast

Lunch

Dinner

Snacks & Dessert

Beverages

- [ ] Juice
- [ ] Tea
- [ ] Water
- [ ] Milk
- [ ] Soft D
- [ ] Coffee
- [ ] Energy

Symptoms

Date: ___ / ___ / ___

Day ___

Sleep

Bed (last night)	___ am / pm
Asleep	___ am / pm
Woke up	___ am / pm
# of Disruptions	___
Total Hours slept	___

Medications

☐ No Change in Meds

☐ Dosage Changed

☐ New Medication

Details ___

Today's Ratings

Scale: 0 = None, 10 = Severe

Pain	___ / 10
Fatigue	___ / 10
Weakness	___ / 10
Stiffness	___ / 10
Anxiety	___ / 10
Depression	___ / 10
Stress	___ / 10
Anger	___ / 10
Brain Fog / Forgetfulness	___ / 10

Pain location(s)

Circle or shade in where your pain is using pen, pencil or highlighters

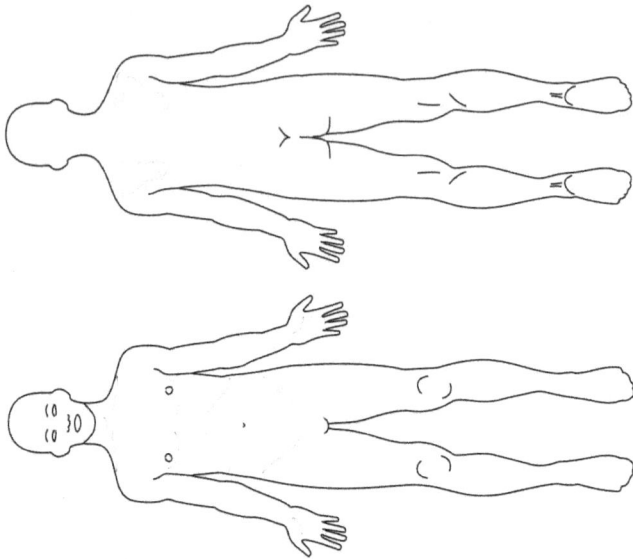

Activity

Active
- [ ] Walking
- [ ] Gym
- [ ] Housework
- [ ] Hydrotherapy

Passive
- [ ] Reading
- [ ] TV
- [ ] Music
- [ ] Light Housework

Meals

Breakfast

Lunch

Dinner

Snacks & Dessert

Beverages
- [ ] Juice
- [ ] Tea
- [ ] Water
- [ ] Milk
- [ ] Soft D
- [ ] Coffee
- [ ] Energy

Symptoms

Date: ____ / ____ / ____   Day ____

Sleep

Bed (last night)	____ am / pm
Asleep	____ am / pm
Woke up	____ am / pm
# of Disruptions	____
Total Hours slept	____

Medications

☐ No Change in Meds
☐ Dosage Changed
☐ New Medication

Details _____

Today's Ratings

Scale: 0 = None, 10 = Severe

Pain	____ /10
Fatigue	____ /10
Weakness	____ /10
Stiffness	____ /10
Anxiety	____ /10
Depression	____ /10
Stress	____ /10
Anger	____ /10
Brain Fog / Forgetfulness	____ /10

Pain location(s)

Circle or shade in where your pain is using pen, pencil or highlighters

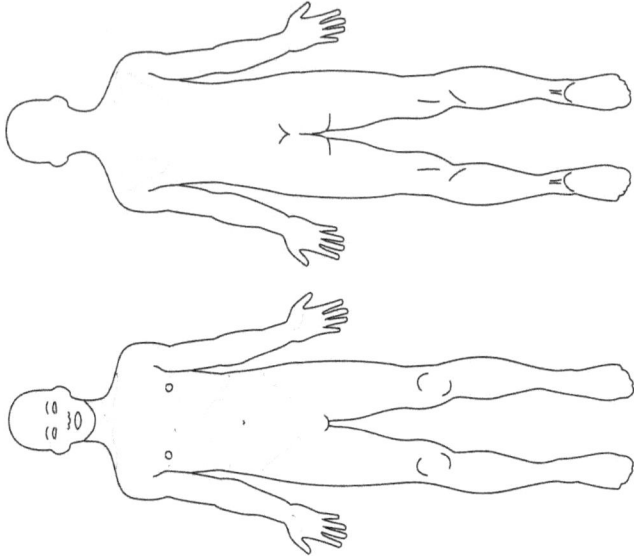

Symptoms

Meals

Breakfast

Lunch

Dinner

Snacks & Dessert

Beverages

☐ Juice ☐ Tea ☐ Water
☐ Milk ☐ Soft D ☐ Coffee
☐ Energy

Activity

Active

☐ Walking ☐ Gym
☐ Housework ☐ Hydrotherapy

Passive

☐ Reading ☐ TV
☐ Music ☐ Light Housework

Date: ___ / ___ / ___

Day ___

Sleep

Bed (last night) _____ am / pm

Asleep _____ am / pm

Woke up _____ am / pm

# of Disruptions _____

Total/Hours slept _____

Today's Ratings

Scale: 0 = None, 10 = Severe

Pain _____ / 10

Fatigue _____ / 10

Weakness _____ / 10

Stiffness _____ / 10

Anxiety _____ / 10

Depression _____ / 10

Stress _____ / 10

Anger _____ / 10

Brain Fog / _____ / 10

Forgetfulness

Medications

☐ No Change in Meds

☐ Dosage Changed

☐ New Medication

Details

Pain location(s)

Circle or shade in where your pain is using pen, pencil or highlighters

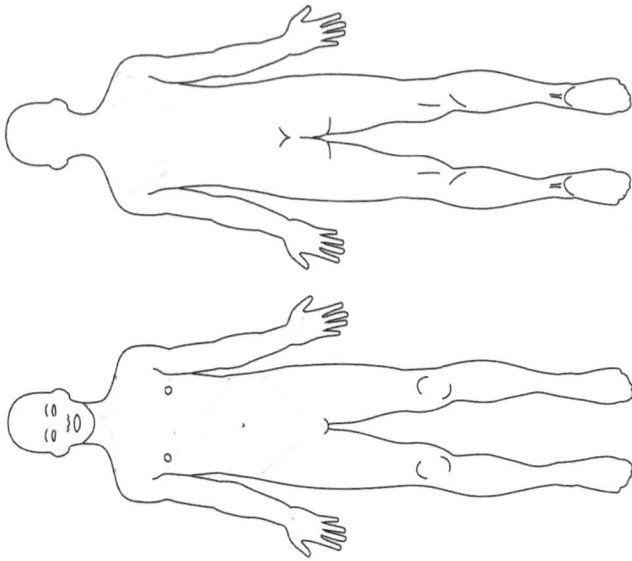

Symptoms

Meals

Breakfast

Lunch

Dinner

Snacks & Dessert

Beverages

- [ ] Juice
- [ ] Tea
- [ ] Water
- [ ] Milk
- [ ] Soft D
- [ ] Coffee
- [ ] Energy

Activity

Active

- [ ] Walking
- [ ] Gym
- [ ] Housework
- [ ] Hydrotherapy

Passive

- [ ] Reading
- [ ] TV
- [ ] Music
- [ ] Light Housework

Date: ___ / ___ / ___   Day ___

Sleep

Bed (last night)	____ am / pm
Asleep	____ am / pm
Woke up	____ am / pm
# of Disruptions	____
Total Hours slept	____

Medications

☐ No Change in Meds

☐ Dosage Changed

☐ New Medication

Details _____

Today's Ratings

Scale: 0 = None, 10 = Severe

Pain	____ / 10
Fatigue	____ / 10
Weakness	____ / 10
Stiffness	____ / 10
Anxiety	____ / 10
Depression	____ / 10
Stress	____ / 10
Anger	____ / 10
Brain Fog / Forgetfulness	____ / 10

Pain location(s)

Circle or shade in where your pain is using pen, pencil or highlighters

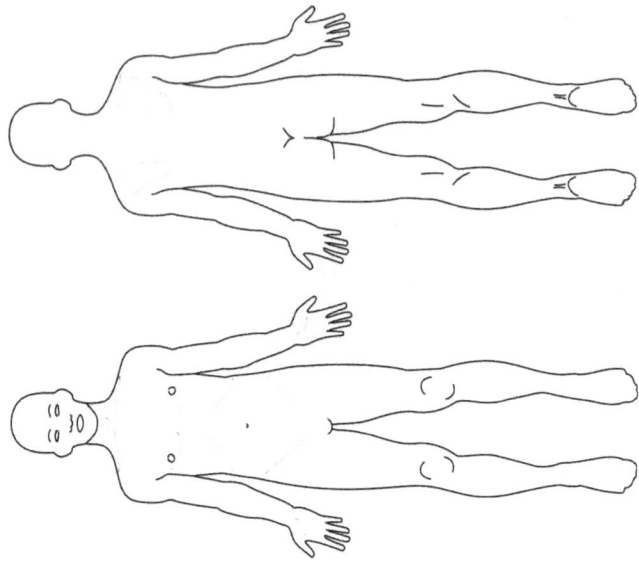

Symptoms

Meals

Breakfast

Lunch

Dinner

Snacks & Dessert

Beverages

☐ Juice ☐ Tea ☐ Water

☐ Milk ☐ Soft D ☐ Coffee

☐ Energy

Activity

Active

☐ Walking ☐ Gym

☐ Housework ☐ Hydrotherapy

Passive

☐ Reading ☐ TV

☐ Music ☐ Light Housework

Date: ___ / ___ / ___   Day ___

Sleep

Bed (last night)	___ am / pm
Asleep	___ am / pm
Woke up	___ am / pm
# of Disruptions	___
Total/Hours slept	___

Medications

☐ No Change in Meds

☐ Dosage Changed

☐ New Medication

Details _____

_____

Today's Ratings

Scale: 0 = None, 10 = Severe

Pain	___ / 10
Fatigue	___ / 10
Weakness	___ / 10
Stiffness	___ / 10
Anxiety	___ / 10
Depression	___ / 10
Stress	___ / 10
Anger	___ / 10
Brain Fog / Forgetfulness	___ / 10

Pain location(s)

Circle or shade in where your pain is using pen, pencil or highlighters

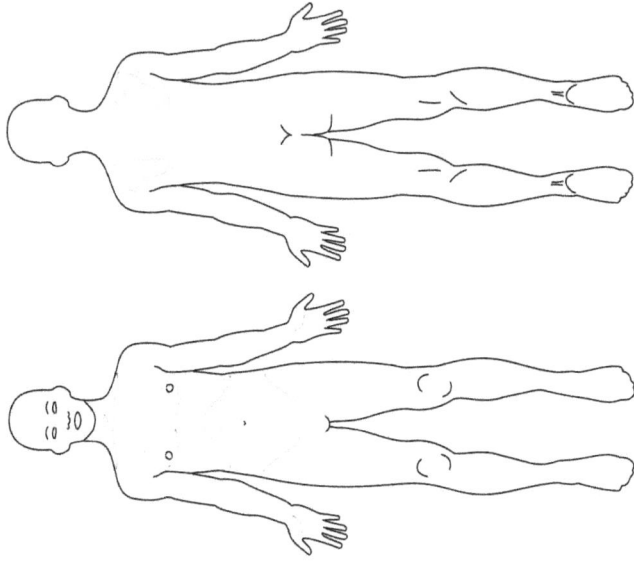

Symptoms

Meals

Breakfast

Lunch

Dinner

Snacks & Dessert

Beverages

☐ Juice ☐ Tea ☐ Water

☐ Milk ☐ Soft D ☐ Coffee

☐ Energy

Activity

Active

☐ Walking ☐ Gym

☐ Housework ☐ Hydrotherapy

Passive

☐ Reading ☐ TV

☐ Music ☐ Light Housework

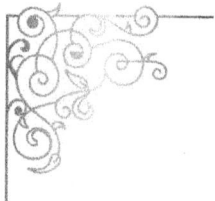

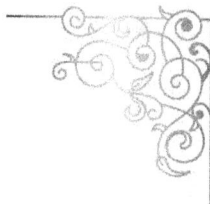

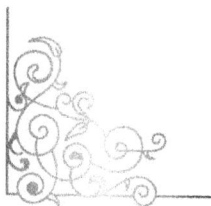

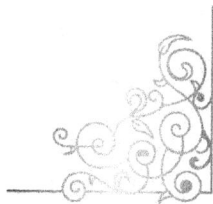

Finding this
Chronic Pain & Fatigue Symtom Diary
helpful?

Don't wait until you run out of pages
before ordering another copy!

ORDER TODAY SO YOU DON'T FORGET

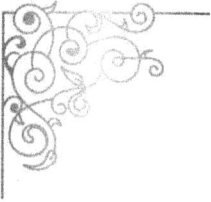

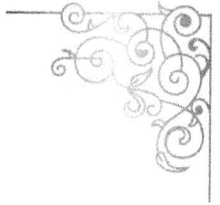

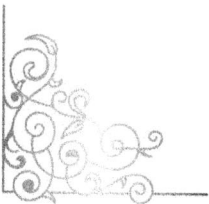

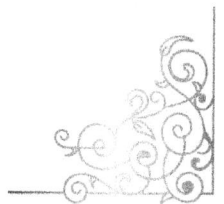

MONTH Three

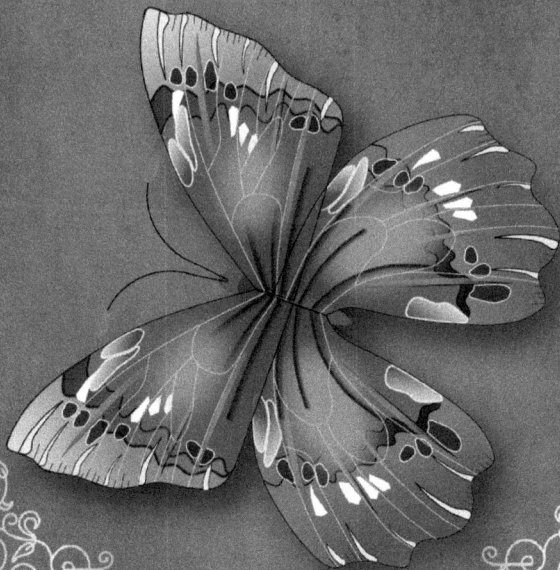

Date: ___ / ___ / ___

Day ___

Sleep

Bed (last night)	___ am / pm
Asleep	___ am / pm
Woke up	___ am / pm
# of Disruptions	___
Total/Hours slept	___

Medications

☐ No Change in Meds

☐ Dosage Changed

☐ New Medication

Details

Today's Ratings

Scale: 0 = None, 10 = Severe

Pain	___ / 10
Fatigue	___ / 10
Weakness	___ / 10
Stiffness	___ / 10
Anxiety	___ / 10
Depression	___ / 10
Stress	___ / 10
Anger	___ / 10
Brain Fog / Forgetfulness	___ / 10

Pain location(s)

Circle or shade in where your pain is using pen, pencil or highlighters

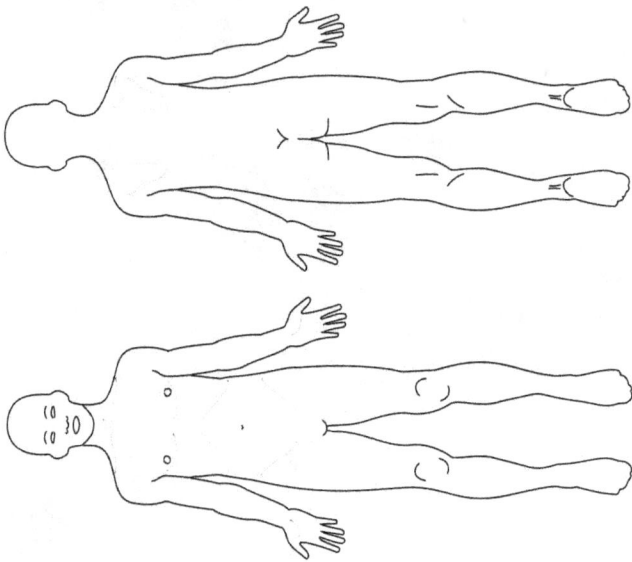

Symptoms

Meals

Breakfast

Lunch

Dinner

Snacks & Dessert

Beverages

☐ Juice   ☐ Tea   ☐ Water
☐ Milk   ☐ Soft D   ☐ Coffee
                       ☐ Energy

Activity

Active

☐ Walking   ☐ Gym
☐ Housework   ☐ Hydrotherapy

Passive

☐ Reading   ☐ TV
☐ Music   ☐ Light Housework

Date: ___ / ___ / ___   Day ___

Sleep

Bed (last night)   ___ am / pm
Asleep   ___ am / pm
Woke up   ___ am / pm
# of Disruptions   ___
Total Hours slept   ___

Medications

☐ No Change in Meds
☐ Dosage Changed
☐ New Medication

Details

Today's Ratings
Scale: 0 = None, 10 = Severe

Pain   ___ / 10
Fatigue   ___ / 10
Weakness   ___ / 10
Stiffness   ___ / 10
Anxiety   ___ / 10
Depression   ___ / 10
Stress   ___ / 10
Anger   ___ / 10
Brain Fog /   ___ / 10
Forgetfulness

Pain location(s)
Circle or shade in where your pain is using pen, pencil or highlighters

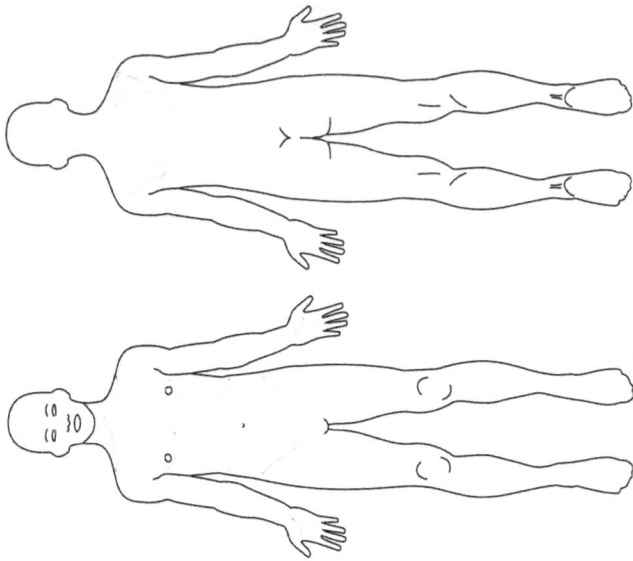

Activity

Active

☐ Walking ☐ Gym
☐ Housework ☐ Hydrotherapy

Passive

☐ Reading ☐ TV
☐ Music ☐ Light Housework

Meals

Breakfast

Lunch

Dinner

Snacks & Dessert

Beverages

☐ Juice ☐ Tea ☐ Water
☐ Milk ☐ Soft D ☐ Coffee
  ☐ Energy

Symptoms

Date: ____ / ____ / ____

Day ____

Sleep

Bed (last night)	_____ am / pm
Asleep	_____ am / pm
Woke up	_____ am / pm
# of Disruptions	_____
Total Hours slept	_____

Medications

☐ No Change in Meds

☐ Dosage Changed

☐ New Medication

Details

Today's Ratings

Scale: 0 = None, 10 = Severe

Pain	____ / 10
Fatigue	____ / 10
Weakness	____ / 10
Stiffness	____ / 10
Anxiety	____ / 10
Depression	____ / 10
Stress	____ / 10
Anger	____ / 10
Brain Fog / Forgetfulness	____ / 10

Pain location(s)

Circle or shade in where your pain is using pen, pencil or highlighters

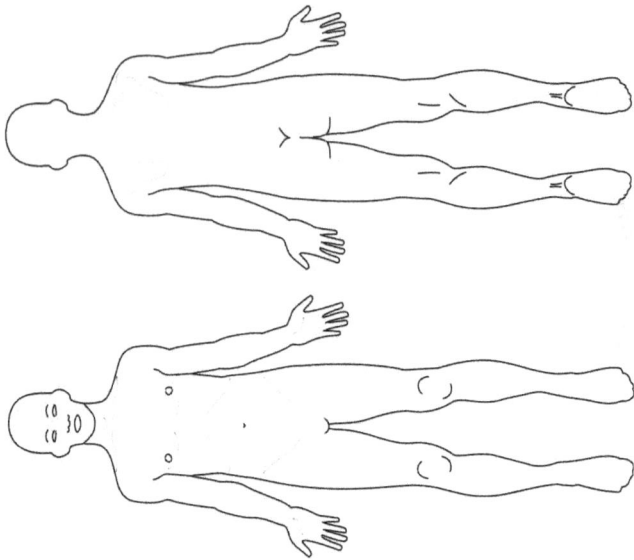

Activity

Active

- [ ] Walking
- [ ] Housework
- [ ] Gym
- [ ] Hydrotherapy

Passive

- [ ] Reading
- [ ] Music
- [ ] TV
- [ ] Light Housework

Meals

Breakfast

Lunch

Dinner

Snacks & Dessert

Beverages

- [ ] Juice
- [ ] Milk
- [ ] Tea
- [ ] Soft D
- [ ] Water
- [ ] Coffee
- [ ] Energy

Symptoms

Date: ___ / ___ / ___   Day ___

Sleep

Bed (last night) _____ am / pm

Asleep _____ am / pm

Woke up _____ am / pm

# of Disruptions _____

Total Hours slept _____

Today's Ratings
Scale: 0 = None, 10 = Severe

Pain _____ /10

Fatigue _____ /10

Weakness _____ /10

Stiffness _____ /10

Anxiety _____ /10

Depression _____ /10

Stress _____ /10

Anger _____ /10

Brain Fog / _____ /10
Forgetfulness

Medications

☐ No Change in Meds

☐ Dosage Changed

☐ New Medication

Details

Pain location(s)

Circle or shade in where your pain is using pen, pencil or highlighters

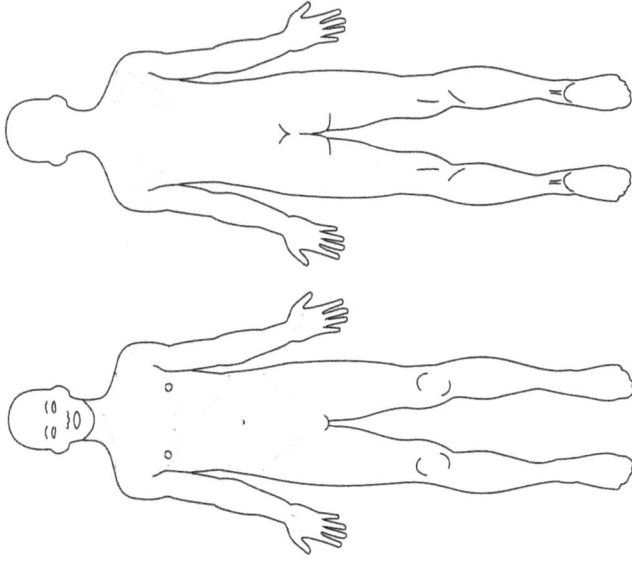

Activity

Active

- [ ] Walking
- [ ] Gym
- [ ] Housework
- [ ] Hydrotherapy

Passive

- [ ] Reading
- [ ] TV
- [ ] Music
- [ ] Light Housework

Meals

Breakfast

Lunch

Dinner

Snacks & Dessert

Beverages

- [ ] Juice
- [ ] Tea
- [ ] Water
- [ ] Milk
- [ ] Soft D
- [ ] Coffee
- [ ] Energy

Symptoms

Date: ____ / ____ / ____   Day ____

Sleep

Bed (last night)	_____ am / pm
Asleep	_____ am / pm
Woke up	_____ am / pm
# of Disruptions	_____
Total Hours slept	_____

Medications

☐ No Change in Meds

☐ Dosage Changed

☐ New Medication

Details

_____

_____

Today's Ratings

Scale: 0 = None, 10 = Severe

Pain	_____ / 10
Fatigue	_____ / 10
Weakness	_____ / 10
Stiffness	_____ / 10
Anxiety	_____ / 10
Depression	_____ / 10
Stress	_____ / 10
Anger	_____ / 10
Brain Fog / Forgetfulness	_____ / 10

Pain location(s)

Circle or shade in where your pain is using pen, pencil or highlighters

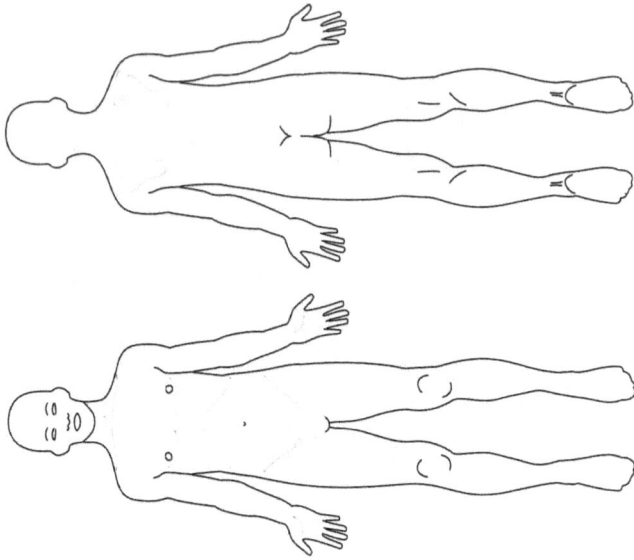

Meals

Symptoms

Breakfast

Lunch

Dinner

Snacks & Dessert

Beverages

☐ Juice ☐ Tea ☐ Water
☐ Milk ☐ Soft D ☐ Coffee
              ☐ Energy

Activity

Active

☐ Walking ☐ Gym
☐ Housework ☐ Hydrotherapy

Passive

☐ Reading ☐ TV
☐ Music ☐ Light Housework

Date: ____ / ___ / ____   Day ____

Sleep

Bed (last night)	____ am / pm
Asleep	____ am / pm
Woke up	____ am / pm
# of Disruptions	____
Total Hours slept	____

Medications

☐ No Change in Meds

☐ Dosage Changed

☐ New Medication

Details

Today's Ratings

Scale: 0 = None, 10 = Severe

Pain	____ / 10
Fatigue	____ / 10
Weakness	____ / 10
Stiffness	____ / 10
Anxiety	____ / 10
Depression	____ / 10
Stress	____ / 10
Anger	____ / 10
Brain Fog / Forgetfulness	____ / 10

Pain location(s)

Circle or shade in where your pain is using pen, pencil or highlighters

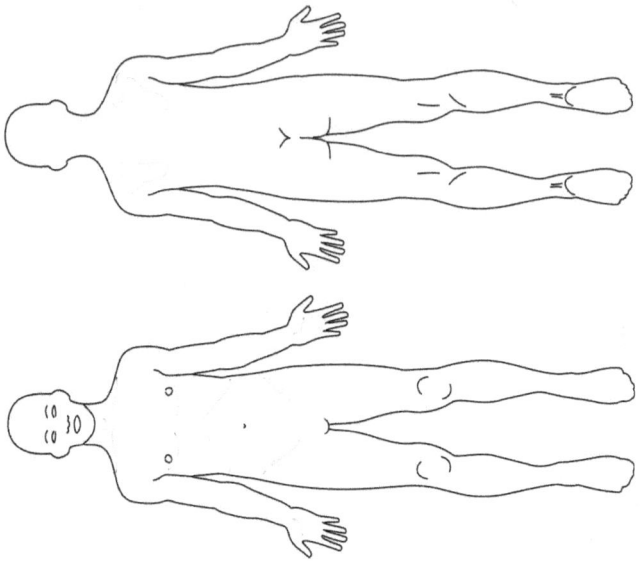

Activity

Active

- [ ] Walking
- [ ] Gym
- [ ] Housework
- [ ] Hydrotherapy

Passive

- [ ] Reading
- [ ] TV
- [ ] Music
- [ ] Light Housework

Meals

Breakfast

Lunch

Dinner

Snacks & Dessert

Beverages

- [ ] Juice
- [ ] Tea
- [ ] Water
- [ ] Milk
- [ ] Soft D
- [ ] Coffee
- [ ] Energy

Symptoms

Date: ___ / ___ / ___   Day ___

Sleep

Bed (last night)	___ am / pm
Asleep	___ am / pm
Woke up	___ am / pm
# of Disruptions	___
Total Hours slept	___

Medications

☐ No Change in Meds
☐ Dosage Changed
☐ New Medication

Details _____

Today's Ratings

Scale: 0 = None, 10 = Severe

Pain	___ /10
Fatigue	___ /10
Weakness	___ /10
Stiffness	___ /10
Anxiety	___ /10
Depression	___ /10
Stress	___ /10
Anger	___ /10
Brain Fog / Forgetfulness	___ /10

Pain location(s)

Circle or shade in where your pain is using pen, pencil or highlighters

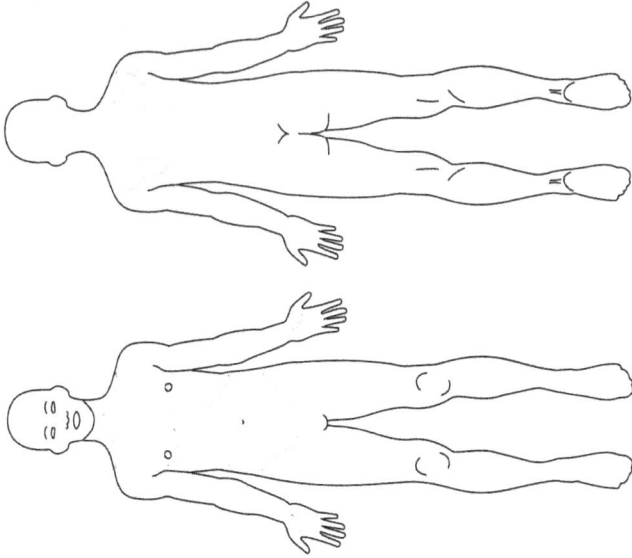

Activity

Active

☐ Walking ☐ Gym
☐ Housework ☐ Hydrotherapy

Passive

☐ Reading ☐ TV
☐ Music ☐ Light Housework

Meals

Breakfast

Lunch

Dinner

Snacks & Dessert

Beverages

☐ Juice ☐ Tea ☐ Water
☐ Milk ☐ Soft D ☐ Coffee
☐ Energy

Symptoms

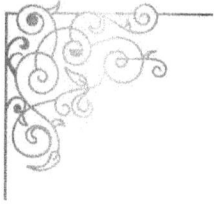

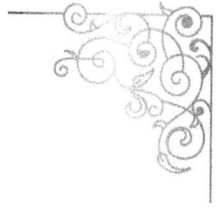

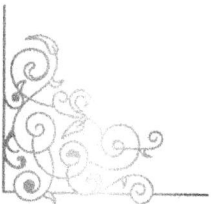

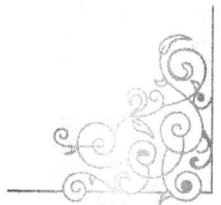

Did you remember to order
another copy of this
Chronic Pain & Fatigue Symtom Diary
last week ?

PUT IT ON YOUR TO DO LIST

Date: ___/___/___

Day ___

Sleep

Bed (last night)	___ am / pm
Asleep	___ am / pm
Woke up	___ am / pm
# of Disruptions	___
Total Hours slept	___

Medications

☐ No Change in Meds

☐ Dosage Changed

☐ New Medication

Details _____

Today's Ratings
Scale: 0 = None, 10 = Severe

Pain	___ / 10
Fatigue	___ / 10
Weakness	___ / 10
Stiffness	___ / 10
Anxiety	___ / 10
Depression	___ / 10
Stress	___ / 10
Anger	___ / 10
Brain Fog / Forgetfulness	___ / 10

Pain location(s)
Circle or shade in where your pain is using pen, pencil or highlighters

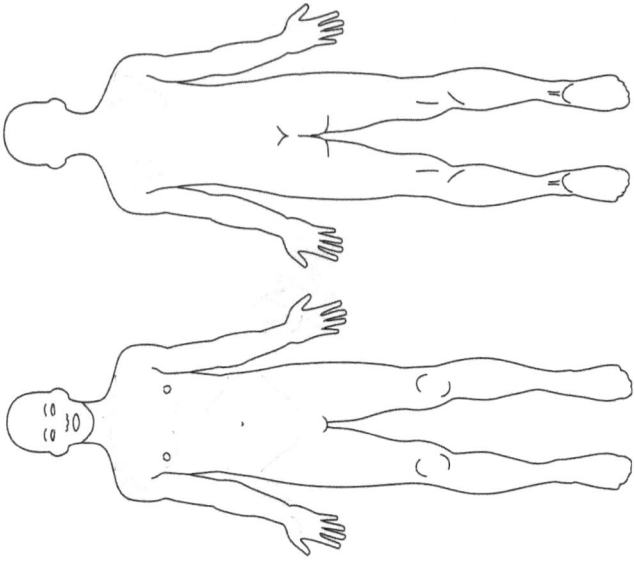

Symptoms

Meals

Breakfast

Lunch

Dinner

Snacks & Dessert

Beverages

- [ ] Juice
- [ ] Tea
- [ ] Water
- [ ] Milk
- [ ] Soft D
- [ ] Coffee
- [ ] Energy

Activity

Active

- [ ] Walking
- [ ] Gym
- [ ] Housework
- [ ] Hydrotherapy

Passive

- [ ] Reading
- [ ] TV
- [ ] Music
- [ ] Light Housework

Date: ___ / ___ / ___   Day ___

Sleep

Bed (last night) _____ am / pm

Asleep _____ am / pm

Woke up _____ am / pm

# of Disruptions _____

Total Hours slept _____

Today's Ratings

Scale: 0 = None, 10 = Severe

Pain _____ / 10

Fatigue _____ / 10

Weakness _____ / 10

Stiffness _____ / 10

Anxiety _____ / 10

Depression _____ / 10

Stress _____ / 10

Anger _____ / 10

Brain Fog / Forgetfulness _____ / 10

Medications

☐ No Change in Meds

☐ Dosage Changed

☐ New Medication

Details

_____

_____

Pain location(s)

Circle or shade in where your pain is using pen, pencil or highlighters

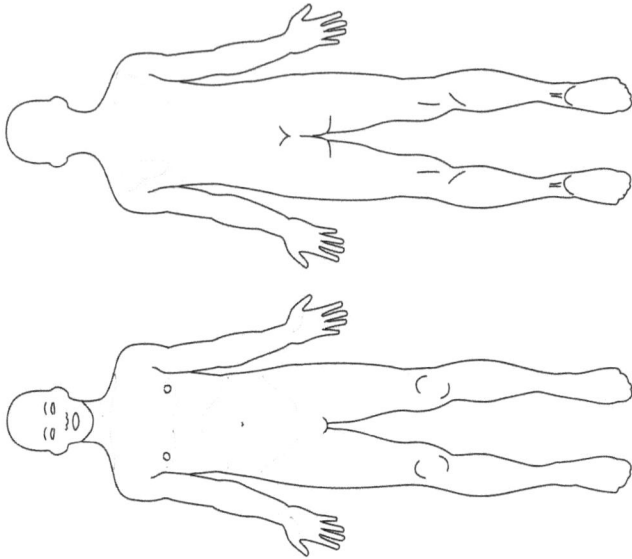

Symptoms

Meals

Breakfast

Lunch

Dinner

Snacks & Dessert

Beverages

- [ ] Juice
- [ ] Milk
- [ ] Tea
- [ ] Soft D
- [ ] Water
- [ ] Coffee
- [ ] Energy

Activity

Active

- [ ] Walking
- [ ] Housework
- [ ] Gym
- [ ] Hydrotherapy

Passive

- [ ] Reading
- [ ] Music
- [ ] TV
- [ ] Light Housework

Date: ___ / ___ / ___   Day ___

Sleep

Bed (last night)	_____ am / pm
Asleep	_____ am / pm
Woke up	_____ am / pm
# of Disruptions	_____
Total hours slept	_____

Medications

☐ No Change in Meds
☐ Dosage Changed
☐ New Medication

Details _____

Today's Ratings

Scale: 0 = None, 10 = Severe

Pain	____ / 10
Fatigue	____ / 10
Weakness	____ / 10
Stiffness	____ / 10
Anxiety	____ / 10
Depression	____ / 10
Stress	____ / 10
Anger	____ / 10
Brain Fog / Forgetfulness	____ / 10

Pain location(s)

Circle or shade in where your pain is using pen, pencil or highlighters

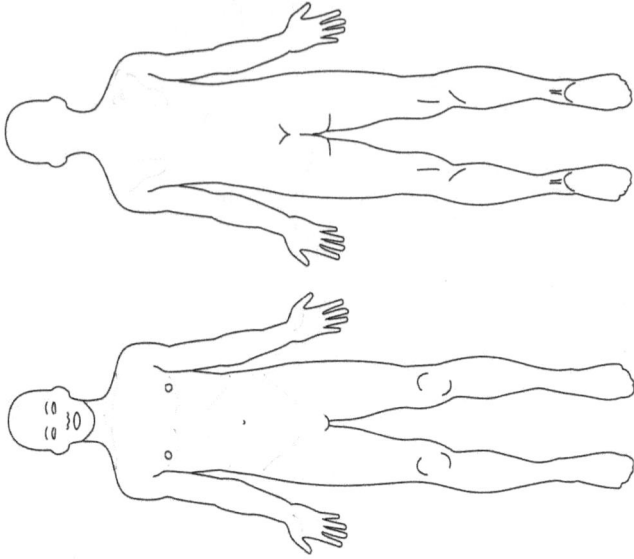

Activity

Active

- [ ] Walking
- [ ] Housework
- [ ] Gym
- [ ] Hydrotherapy

Passive

- [ ] Reading
- [ ] Music
- [ ] TV
- [ ] Light Housework

Meals

Breakfast

Lunch

Dinner

Snacks & Dessert

Beverages

- [ ] Juice
- [ ] Milk
- [ ] Tea
- [ ] Soft D
- [ ] Water
- [ ] Coffee
- [ ] Energy

Symptoms

Date: _____ / _____ / _____   Day _____

Sleep

Bed (last night)	_____ am / pm
Asleep	_____ am / pm
Woke up	_____ am / pm
# of Disruptions	_____
Total Hours slept	_____

Medications

☐ No Change in Meds

☐ Dosage Changed

☐ New Medication

Details _____

_____

Today's Ratings

Scale: 0 = None, 10 = Severe

Pain	_____ / 10
Fatigue	_____ / 10
Weakness	_____ / 10
Stiffness	_____ / 10
Anxiety	_____ / 10
Depression	_____ / 10
Stress	_____ / 10
Anger	_____ / 10
Brain Fog / Forgetfulness	_____ / 10

Pain location(s)

Circle or shade in where your pain is using pen, pencil or highlighters

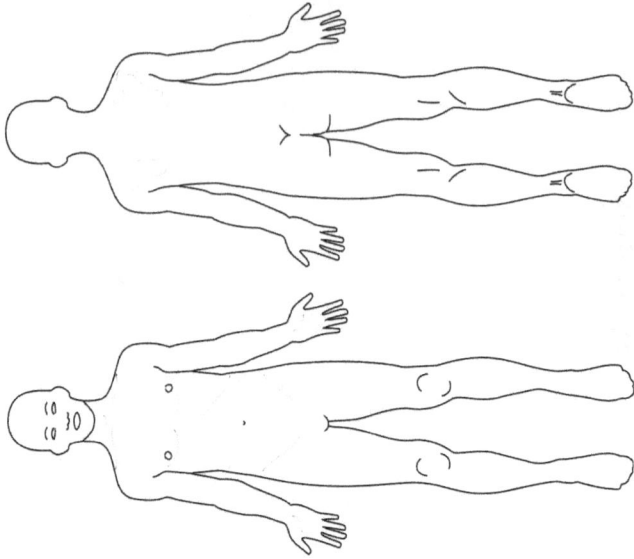

Symptoms

Meals

Breakfast

Lunch

Dinner

Snacks & Dessert

Beverages

- [ ] Juice
- [ ] Milk
- [ ] Tea
- [ ] Soft D
- [ ] Water
- [ ] Coffee
- [ ] Energy

Activity

Active

- [ ] Walking
- [ ] Housework
- [ ] Gym
- [ ] Hydrotherapy

Passive

- [ ] Reading
- [ ] Music
- [ ] TV
- [ ] Light Housework

Date: ____ / ____ / ____   Day ____

Sleep

Bed (last night)	____ am / pm
Asleep	____ am / pm
Woke up	____ am / pm
# of Disruptions	____
Total Hours slept	____

Medications

☐ No Change in Meds

☐ Dosage Changed

☐ New Medication

Details

Today's Ratings

Scale: 0 = None, 10 = Severe

Pain	____ / 10
Fatigue	____ / 10
Weakness	____ / 10
Stiffness	____ / 10
Anxiety	____ / 10
Depression	____ / 10
Stress	____ / 10
Anger	____ / 10
Brain Fog / Forgetfulness	____ / 10

Pain location(s)

Circle or shade in where your pain is using pen, pencil or highlighters

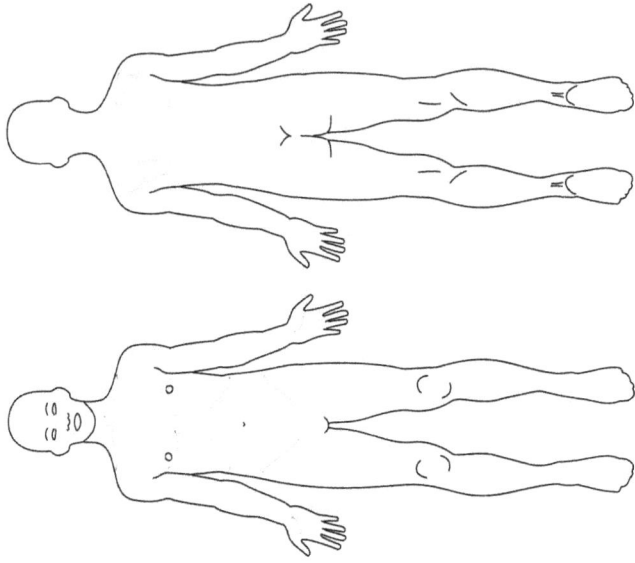

Activity

Active

- [ ] Walking
- [ ] Housework
- [ ] Gym
- [ ] Hydrotherapy

Passive

- [ ] Reading
- [ ] Music
- [ ] TV
- [ ] Light Housework

Meals

Breakfast

Lunch

Dinner

Snacks & Dessert

Beverages

- [ ] Juice
- [ ] Milk
- [ ] Tea
- [ ] Soft D
- [ ] Water
- [ ] Coffee
- [ ] Energy

Symptoms

Date: _____ / _____ / _____   Day _____

Sleep

Bed (last night)	_____	am / pm
Asleep	_____	am / pm
Woke up	_____	am / pm
# of Disruptions	_____	
Total/Hours slept	_____	

Medications

☐ No Change in Meds

☐ Dosage Changed

☐ New Medication

Details

_____

_____

Today's Ratings

Scale: 0 = None, 10 = Severe

Pain	_____ / 10
Fatigue	_____ / 10
Weakness	_____ / 10
Stiffness	_____ / 10
Anxiety	_____ / 10
Depression	_____ / 10
Stress	_____ / 10
Anger	_____ / 10
Brain Fog / Forgetfulness	_____ / 10

Pain location(s)

Circle or shade in where your pain is using pen, pencil or highlighters

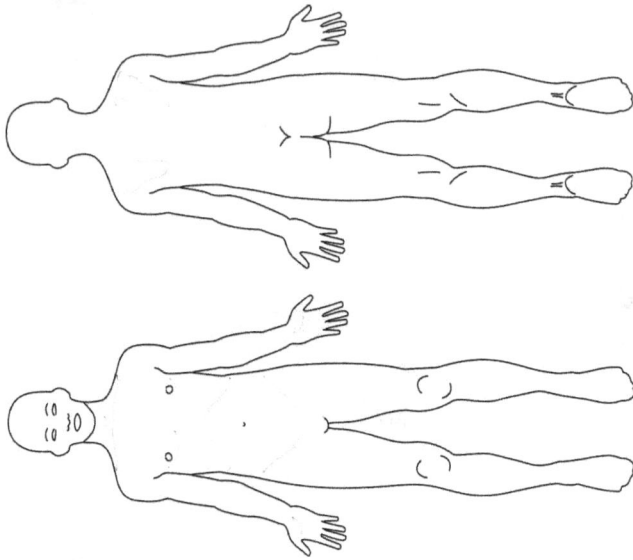

Activity

Active

- [ ] Walking
- [ ] Gym
- [ ] Housework
- [ ] Hydrotherapy

Passive

- [ ] Reading
- [ ] TV
- [ ] Music
- [ ] Light Housework

Meals

Breakfast

Lunch

Dinner

Snacks & Dessert

Beverages

- [ ] Juice
- [ ] Tea
- [ ] Water
- [ ] Milk
- [ ] Soft D
- [ ] Coffee
- [ ] Energy

Symptoms

Date: _____ / _____ / _____   Day _____

Sleep

Bed (last night) _____ am / pm

Asleep _____ am / pm

Woke up _____ am / pm

# of Disruptions _____

Total/Hours slept _____

Medications

☐ No Change in Meds

☐ Dosage Changed

☐ New Medication

Details

Today's Ratings

Scale: 0 = None, 10 = Severe

Pain	_____ / 10
Fatigue	_____ / 10
Weakness	_____ / 10
Stiffness	_____ / 10
Anxiety	_____ / 10
Depression	_____ / 10
Stress	_____ / 10
Anger	_____ / 10
Brain Fog /	_____ / 10
Forgetfulness	

Pain location(s)

Circle or shade in where your pain is using pen, pencil or highlighters

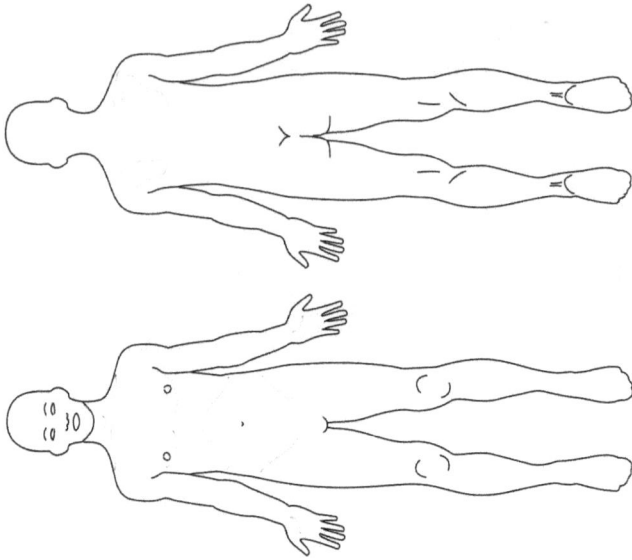

Activity

Active

☐ Walking   ☐ Gym

☐ Housework   ☐ Hydrotherapy

Passive

☐ Reading   ☐ TV

☐ Music   ☐ Light Housework

Meals

Breakfast

Lunch

Dinner

Snacks & Dessert

Beverages

☐ Juice   ☐ Tea   ☐ Water

☐ Milk   ☐ Soft D   ☐ Coffee

   ☐ Energy

Symptoms

Date: ____ / ____ / ____   Day ____

Sleep

Bed (last night)	_____ am / pm
Asleep	_____ am / pm
Woke up	_____ am / pm
# of Disruptions	_____
Total Hours slept	_____

Medications

☐ No Change in Meds

☐ Dosage Changed

☐ New Medication

Details _____

Today's Ratings

Scale: 0 = None, 10 = Severe

Pain	_____ / 10
Fatigue	_____ / 10
Weakness	_____ / 10
Stiffness	_____ / 10
Anxiety	_____ / 10
Depression	_____ / 10
Stress	_____ / 10
Anger	_____ / 10
Brain Fog / Forgetfulness	_____ / 10

Pain location(s)

Circle or shade in where your pain is using pen, pencil or highlighters

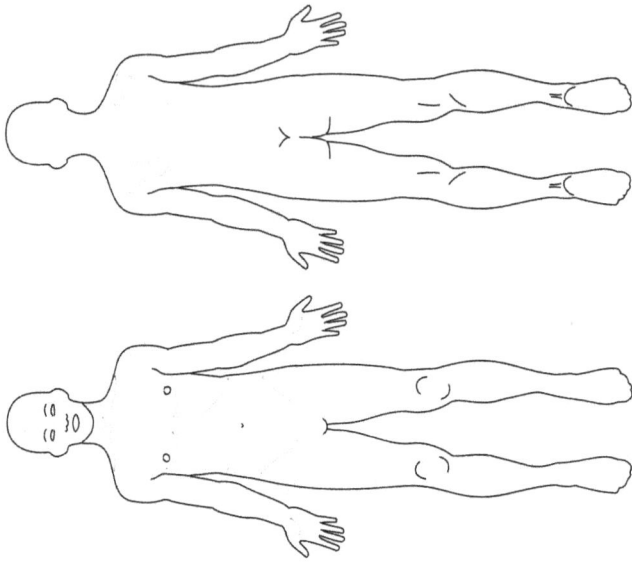

Activity

Active

- [ ] Walking
- [ ] Gym
- [ ] Housework
- [ ] Hydrotherapy

Passive

- [ ] Reading
- [ ] TV
- [ ] Music
- [ ] Light Housework

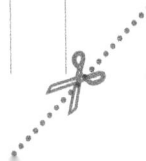

Meals

Breakfast

Lunch

Dinner

Snacks & Dessert

Beverages

- [ ] Juice
- [ ] Tea
- [ ] Water
- [ ] Milk
- [ ] Soft D
- [ ] Coffee
- [ ] Energy

Symptoms

Date: ____ / ____ / ____   Day ____

Sleep

Bed (last night) _____ am / pm

Asleep _____ am / pm

Woke up _____ am / pm

# of Disruptions _____

Total/Hours slept _____

Medications

☐ No Change in Meds

☐ Dosage Changed

☐ New Medication

Details _____

_____

Today's Ratings
Scale: 0 = None, 10 = Severe

Pain _____ / 10

Fatigue _____ / 10

Weakness _____ / 10

Stiffness _____ / 10

Anxiety _____ / 10

Depression _____ / 10

Stress _____ / 10

Anger _____ / 10

Brain Fog / _____ / 10
Forgetfulness

Pain location(s)
Circle or shade in where your pain is using pen, pencil or highlighters

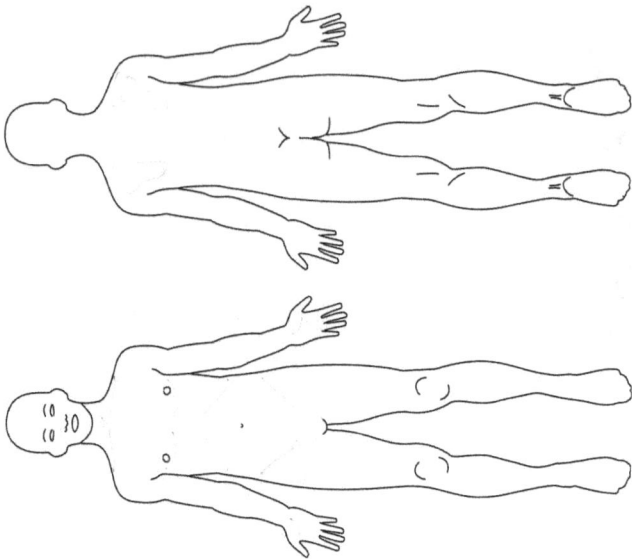

Activity

Active

☐ Walking ☐ Gym
☐ Housework ☐ Hydrotherapy

Passive

☐ Reading ☐ TV
☐ Music ☐ Light Housework

Meals

Breakfast

Lunch

Dinner

Snacks & Dessert

Beverages

☐ Juice ☐ Tea ☐ Water
☐ Milk ☐ Soft D ☐ Coffee
☐ Energy

Symptoms

Date: ____ / ____ / ____

Day ____

Sleep

Bed (last night) _____ am / pm

Asleep _____ am / pm

Woke up _____ am / pm

# of Disruptions _____

Total Hours slept _____

Medications

☐ No Change in Meds

☐ Dosage Changed

☐ New Medication

Details _____

_____

Today's Ratings

Scale: 0 = None, 10 = Severe

Pain _____ / 10

Fatigue _____ / 10

Weakness _____ / 10

Stiffness _____ / 10

Anxiety _____ / 10

Depression _____ / 10

Stress _____ / 10

Anger _____ / 10

Brain Fog / _____ / 10
Forgetfulness

Pain location(s)

Circle or shade in where your pain is using pen, pencil or highlighters

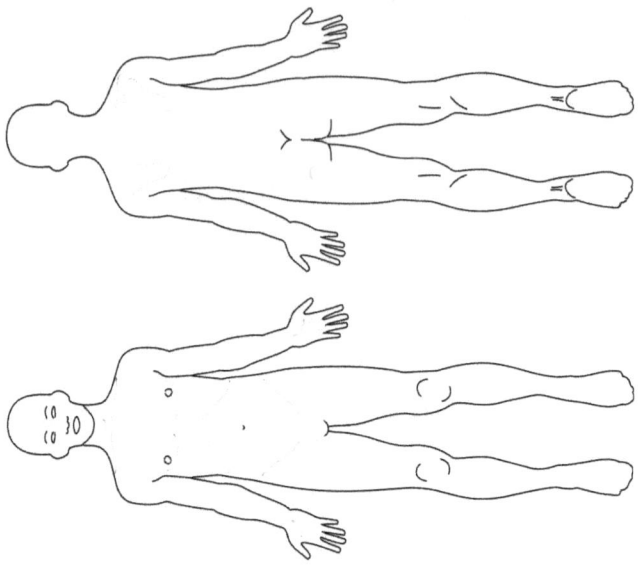

Symptoms

Meals

Breakfast

Lunch

Dinner

Snacks & Dessert

Beverages

☐ Juice ☐ Tea ☐ Water
☐ Milk ☐ Soft D ☐ Coffee
                    ☐ Energy

Activity

Active

☐ Walking ☐ Gym
☐ Housework ☐ Hydrotherapy

Passive

☐ Reading ☐ TV
☐ Music ☐ Light Housework

Date: ____ / ____ / ____

Day ____

Sleep

Bed (last night) _____ am / pm

Asleep _____ am / pm

Woke up _____ am / pm

# of Disruptions _____

Total/Hours slept _____

Medications

☐ No Change in Meds

☐ Dosage Changed

☐ New Medication

Details

_____

_____

Today's Ratings

Scale: 0 = None, 10 = Severe

Pain _____ / 10

Fatigue _____ / 10

Weakness _____ / 10

Stiffness _____ / 10

Anxiety _____ / 10

Depression _____ / 10

Stress _____ / 10

Anger _____ / 10

Brain Fog / Forgetfulness _____ / 10

Pain location(s)

Circle or shade in where your pain is using pen, pencil or highlighters

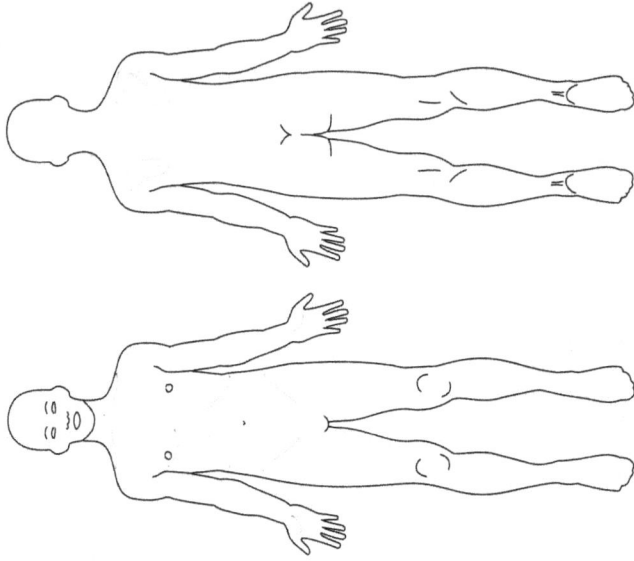

Activity

Active

☐ Walking ☐ Gym
☐ Housework ☐ Hydrotherapy

_____
_____
_____
_____

Passive

☐ Reading ☐ TV
☐ Music ☐ Light Housework

_____
_____
_____

Meals

Breakfast

_____
_____

Lunch

_____
_____

Dinner

_____
_____

Snacks & Dessert

_____
_____

Beverages

☐ Juice ☐ Tea ☐ Water
☐ Milk ☐ Soft D ☐ Coffee
☐ Energy

Symptoms

_____
_____
_____
_____
_____
_____
_____
_____
_____
_____
_____

Date: ____ / ____ / ____

Day ____

Sleep

Bed (last night) _____ am / pm

Asleep _____ am / pm

Woke up _____ am / pm

# of Disruptions _____

Total Hours slept _____

Medications

☐ No Change in Meds

☐ Dosage Changed

☐ New Medication

Details _____

_____

Today's Ratings
Scale: 0 = None, 10 = Severe

Pain _____ / 10

Fatigue _____ / 10

Weakness _____ / 10

Stiffness _____ / 10

Anxiety _____ / 10

Depression _____ / 10

Stress _____ / 10

Anger _____ / 10

Brain Fog /
Forgetfulness _____ / 10

Pain location(s)
Circle or shade in where your pain is using pen, pencil or highlighters

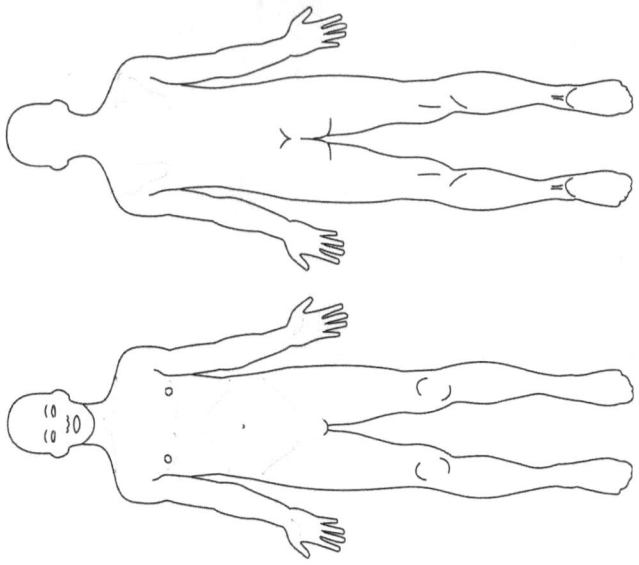

Activity

Active

- [ ] Walking
- [ ] Gym
- [ ] Housework
- [ ] Hydrotherapy

Passive

- [ ] Reading
- [ ] TV
- [ ] Music
- [ ] Light Housework

Meals

Breakfast

Lunch

Dinner

Snacks & Dessert

Beverages

- [ ] Juice
- [ ] Tea
- [ ] Water
- [ ] Milk
- [ ] Soft D
- [ ] Coffee
- [ ] Energy

Symptoms

Date: _____ / _____ / _____   Day _____

Sleep

Bed (last night)	_____ am / pm
Asleep	_____ am / pm
Woke up	_____ am / pm
# of Disruptions	_____
Total/Hours slept	_____

Medications

☐ No Change in Meds

☐ Dosage Changed

☐ New Medication

Details _____

_____

Today's Ratings

Scale: 0 = None, 10 = Severe

Pain	_____ / 10
Fatigue	_____ / 10
Weakness	_____ / 10
Stiffness	_____ / 10
Anxiety	_____ / 10
Depression	_____ / 10
Stress	_____ / 10
Anger	_____ / 10
Brain Fog / Forgetfulness	_____ / 10

Pain location(s)

Circle or shade in where your pain is using pen, pencil or highlighters

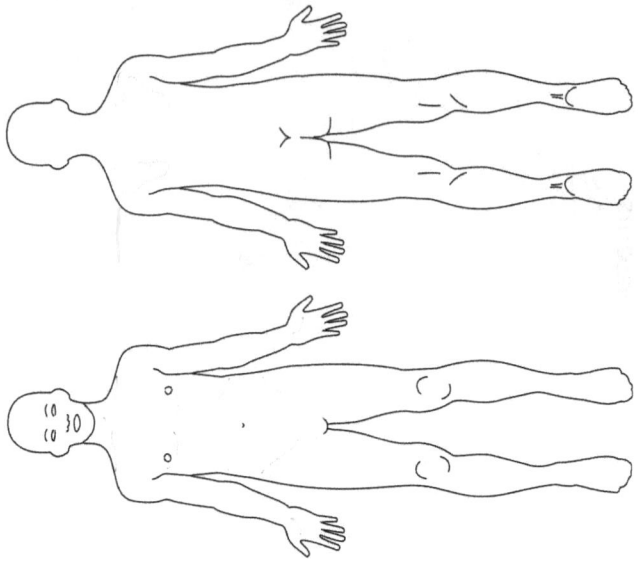

Symptoms

Meals

Breakfast

Lunch

Dinner

Snacks & Dessert

Beverages

- [ ] Juice
- [ ] Milk
- [ ] Tea
- [ ] Soft D
- [ ] Water
- [ ] Coffee
- [ ] Energy

Activity

Active

- [ ] Walking
- [ ] Housework
- [ ] Gym
- [ ] Hydrotherapy

Passive

- [ ] Reading
- [ ] Music
- [ ] TV
- [ ] Light Housework

Date: ___ / ___ / ___   Day ___

Sleep

Bed (last night)	___ am / pm
Asleep	___ am / pm
Woke up	___ am / pm
# of Disruptions	___
Total Hours slept	___

Medications

☐ No Change in Meds

☐ Dosage Changed

☐ New Medication

Details

_____

Today's Ratings

Scale: 0 = None, 10 = Severe

Pain	___ / 10
Fatigue	___ / 10
Weakness	___ / 10
Stiffness	___ / 10
Anxiety	___ / 10
Depression	___ / 10
Stress	___ / 10
Anger	___ / 10
Brain Fog / Forgetfulness	___ / 10

Pain location(s)

Circle or shade in where your pain is using pen, pencil or highlighters

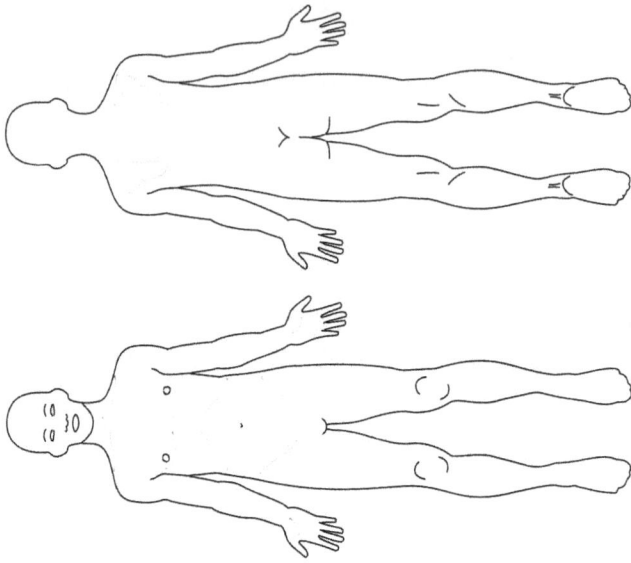

Activity

Active

- [ ] Walking
- [ ] Gym
- [ ] Housework
- [ ] Hydrotherapy

Passive

- [ ] Reading
- [ ] TV
- [ ] Music
- [ ] Light Housework

Meals

Breakfast

Lunch

Dinner

Snacks & Dessert

Beverages

- [ ] Juice
- [ ] Tea
- [ ] Water
- [ ] Milk
- [ ] Soft D
- [ ] Coffee
- [ ] Energy

Symptoms

Date: ___ / ___ / ___   Day ___

Sleep

Bed (last night)   _____ am / pm

Asleep   _____ am / pm

Woke up   _____ am / pm

# of Disruptions   _____

Total Hours slept _____

Medications

☐ No Change in Meds

☐ Dosage Changed

☐ New Medication

Details
_____

Today's Ratings

Scale: 0 = None, 10 = Severe

Pain	_____ / 10
Fatigue	_____ / 10
Weakness	_____ / 10
Stiffness	_____ / 10
Anxiety	_____ / 10
Depression	_____ / 10
Stress	_____ / 10
Anger	_____ / 10
Brain Fog / Forgetfulness	_____ / 10

Pain location(s)

Circle or shade in where your pain is using pen, pencil or highlighters

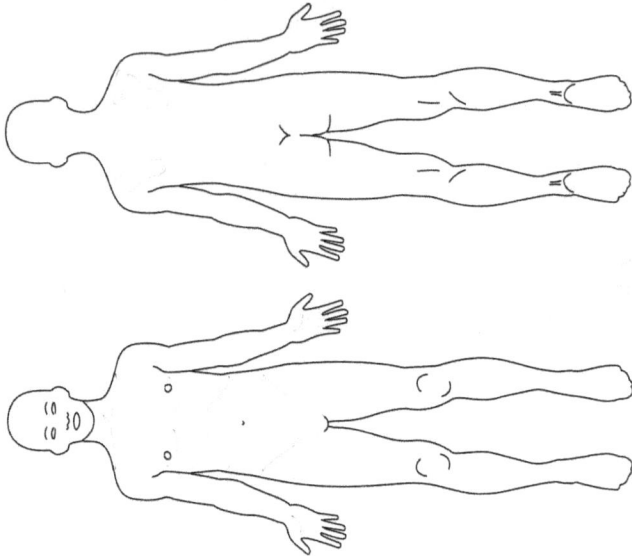

Activity

Active

☐ Walking ☐ Gym
☐ Housework ☐ Hydrotherapy

Passive

☐ Reading ☐ TV
☐ Music ☐ Light Housework

Meals

Breakfast

Lunch

Dinner

Snacks & Dessert

Beverages

☐ Juice ☐ Tea ☐ Water
☐ Milk ☐ Soft D ☐ Coffee
☐ Energy

Symptoms

Date: _____ / _____ / _____

Day _____

Sleep

Bed (last night) _____ am / pm

Asleep _____ am / pm

Woke up _____ am / pm

# of Disruptions _____

Total Hours slept _____

Today's Ratings

Scale: 0 = None, 10 = Severe

Pain	_____ / 10
Fatigue	_____ / 10
Weakness	_____ / 10
Stiffness	_____ / 10
Anxiety	_____ / 10
Depression	_____ / 10
Stress	_____ / 10
Anger	_____ / 10
Brain Fog / Forgetfulness	_____ / 10

Medications

☐ No Change in Meds

☐ Dosage Changed

☐ New Medication

Details _____

_____

Pain location(s)

Circle or shade in where your pain is using pen, pencil or highlighters

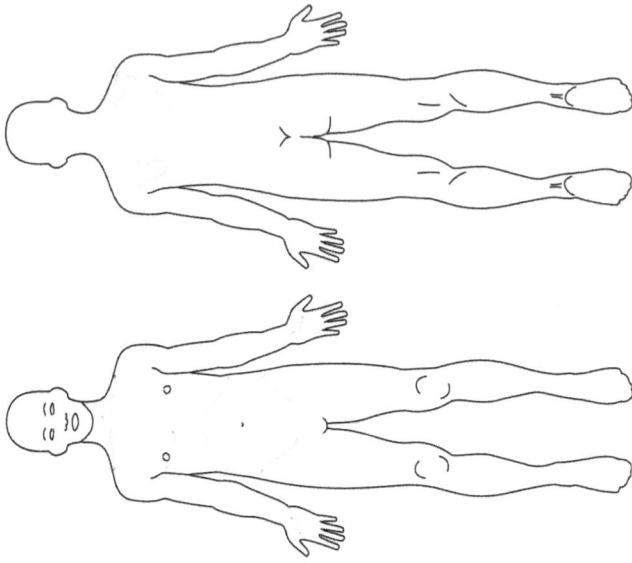

Symptoms

Meals

Breakfast

Lunch

Dinner

Snacks & Dessert

Beverages

- [ ] Juice
- [ ] Milk
- [ ] Tea
- [ ] Soft D
- [ ] Water
- [ ] Coffee
- [ ] Energy

Activity

Active

- [ ] Walking
- [ ] Housework
- [ ] Gym
- [ ] Hydrotherapy

Passive

- [ ] Reading
- [ ] Music
- [ ] TV
- [ ] Light Housework

Date: ____ / ____ / ____

Day ____

Sleep

Bed (last night) _____ am / pm

Asleep _____ am / pm

Woke up _____ am / pm

# of Disruptions _____

Total Hours slept _____

Medications

☐ No Change in Meds

☐ Dosage Changed

☐ New Medication

Details

Today's Ratings

Scale: 0 = None, 10 = Severe

Pain _____ / 10

Fatigue _____ / 10

Weakness _____ / 10

Stiffness _____ / 10

Anxiety _____ / 10

Depression _____ / 10

Stress _____ / 10

Anger _____ / 10

Brain Fog / Forgetfulness _____ / 10

Pain location(s)

Circle or shade in where your pain is using pen, pencil or highlighters

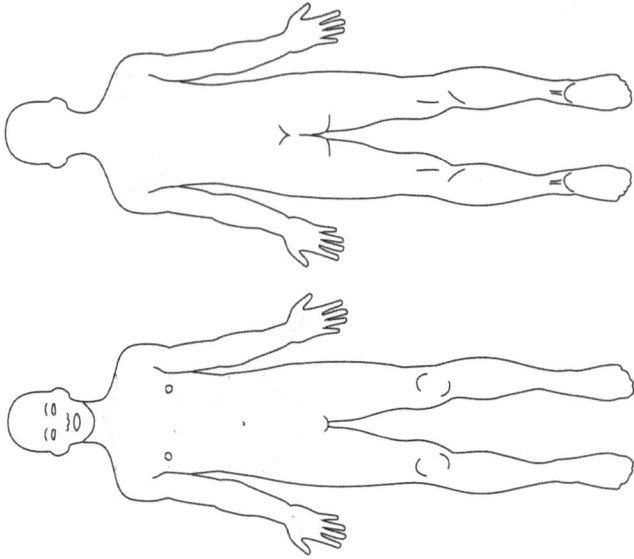

Activity

Active

☐ Walking ☐ Gym
☐ Housework ☐ Hydrotherapy

Passive

☐ Reading ☐ TV
☐ Music ☐ Light Housework

Meals

Breakfast

Lunch

Dinner

Snacks & Dessert

Beverages

☐ Juice ☐ Tea ☐ Water
☐ Milk ☐ Soft D ☐ Coffee
☐ Energy

Symptoms

Date: _____ / _____ / _____   Day _____

Sleep

Bed (last night) _____ am / pm

Asleep _____ am / pm

Woke up _____ am / pm

# of Disruptions _____

Total Hours slept _____

Medications

☐ No Change in Meds

☐ Dosage Changed

☐ New Medication

Details _____

_____

Today's Ratings

Scale: 0 = None, 10 = Severe

Pain _____ / 10

Fatigue _____ / 10

Weakness _____ / 10

Stiffness _____ / 10

Anxiety _____ / 10

Depression _____ / 10

Stress _____ / 10

Anger _____ / 10

Brain Fog / _____ / 10
Forgetfulness

Pain location(s)

Circle or shade in where your pain is using pen, pencil or highlighters

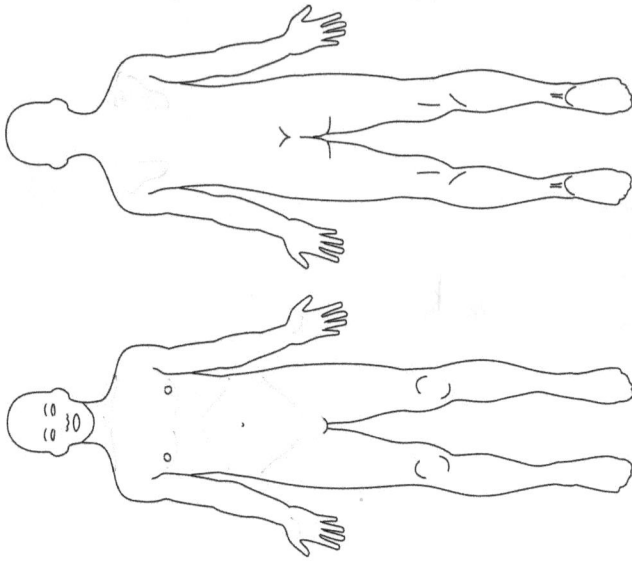

Activity

Active
☐ Walking ☐ Gym
☐ Housework ☐ Hydrotherapy

Passive
☐ Reading ☐ TV
☐ Music ☐ Light Housework

Meals

Breakfast

Lunch

Dinner

Snacks & Dessert

Beverages
☐ Juice ☐ Tea ☐ Water
☐ Milk ☐ Soft D ☐ Coffee
☐ Energy

Symptoms

Date: ____ / ____ / ____

Day ____

Sleep

Bed (last night) _____ am / pm

Asleep _____ am / pm

Woke up _____ am / pm

# of Disruptions _____

Total Hours slept _____

Medications

☐ No Change in Meds

☐ Dosage Changed

☐ New Medication

Details _____

_____

Today's Ratings

Scale: 0 = None, 10 = Severe

Pain _____ / 10

Fatigue _____ / 10

Weakness _____ / 10

Stiffness _____ / 10

Anxiety _____ / 10

Depression _____ / 10

Stress _____ / 10

Anger _____ / 10

Brain Fog / _____ / 10
Forgetfulness

Pain location(s)

Circle or shade in where your pain is using pen, pencil or highlighters

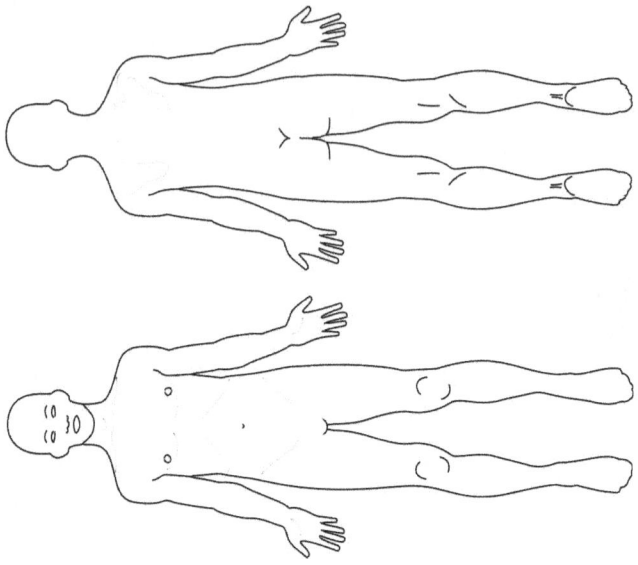

Symptoms

Meals

Breakfast

Lunch

Dinner

Snacks & Dessert

Beverages

☐ Juice   ☐ Tea   ☐ Water
☐ Milk   ☐ Soft D   ☐ Coffee
                          ☐ Energy

Activity

Active

☐ Walking   ☐ Gym
☐ Housework   ☐ Hydrotherapy

Passive

☐ Reading   ☐ TV
☐ Music   ☐ Light Housework

Date: ___ / ___ / ___

Day ___

Sleep

Bed (last night)	___ am / pm
Asleep	___ am / pm
Woke up	___ am / pm
# of Disruptions	___
Total Hours slept	___

Medications

☐ No Change in Meds

☐ Dosage Changed

☐ New Medication

Details _____

Today's Ratings

Scale: 0 = None, 10 = Severe

Pain	___ / 10
Fatigue	___ / 10
Weakness	___ / 10
Stiffness	___ / 10
Anxiety	___ / 10
Depression	___ / 10
Stress	___ / 10
Anger	___ / 10
Brain Fog / Forgetfulness	___ / 10

Pain location(s)

Circle or shade in where your pain is using pen, pencil or highlighters

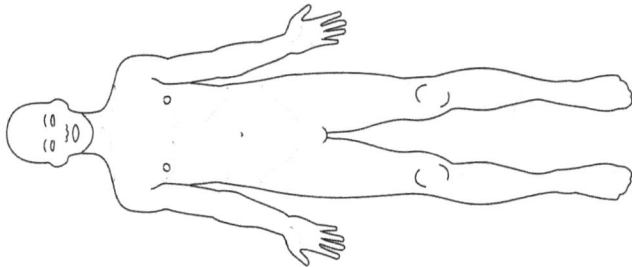

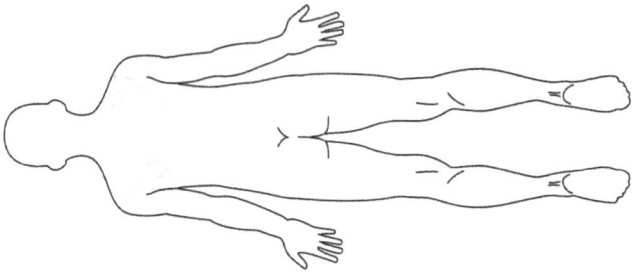

Symptoms

Meals

Breakfast

Lunch

Dinner

Snacks & Dessert

Beverages

☐ Juice ☐ Tea ☐ Water

☐ Milk ☐ Soft D ☐ Coffee

☐ Energy

Activity

Active

☐ Walking ☐ Gym

☐ Housework ☐ Hydrotherapy

Passive

☐ Reading ☐ TV

☐ Music ☐ Light Housework

Date: ___ / ___ / ___   Day ___

Sleep

Bed (last night) _____ am / pm

Asleep _____ am / pm

Woke up _____ am / pm

# of Disruptions _____

Total Hours slept _____

Medications

☐ No Change in Meds

☐ Dosage Changed

☐ New Medication

Details _____

_____

Today's Ratings
Scale: 0 = None, 10 = Severe

Pain	___ / 10
Fatigue	___ / 10
Weakness	___ / 10
Stiffness	___ / 10
Anxiety	___ / 10
Depression	___ / 10
Stress	___ / 10
Anger	___ / 10
Brain Fog / Forgetfulness	___ / 10

Pain location(s)

Circle or shade in where your pain is using pen, pencil or highlighters

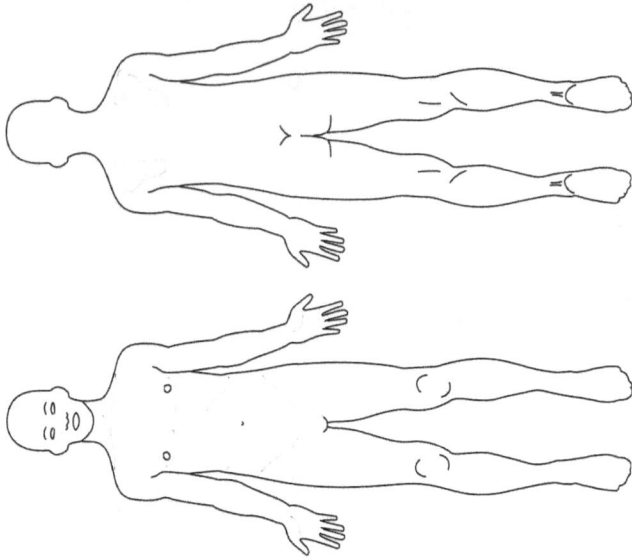

Symptoms

Meals

Breakfast

Lunch

Dinner

Snacks & Dessert

Beverages

- [ ] Juice
- [ ] Milk
- [ ] Tea
- [ ] Soft D
- [ ] Water
- [ ] Coffee
- [ ] Energy

Activity

Active

- [ ] Walking
- [ ] Housework
- [ ] Gym
- [ ] Hydrotherapy

Passive

- [ ] Reading
- [ ] Music
- [ ] TV
- [ ] Light Housework

Date: _____ / _____ / _____   Day _____

Sleep

Bed (last night) _____ am / pm

Asleep _____ am / pm

Woke up _____ am / pm

# of Disruptions _____

Total/Hours slept _____

Medications

☐ No Change in Meds

☐ Dosage Changed

☐ New Medication

Details

Today's Ratings

Scale: 0 = None, 10 = Severe

Pain _____ / 10

Fatigue _____ / 10

Weakness _____ / 10

Stiffness _____ / 10

Anxiety _____ / 10

Depression _____ / 10

Stress _____ / 10

Anger _____ / 10

Brain Fog / _____ / 10
Forgetfulness

Pain location(s)

Circle or shade in where your pain is using pen, pencil or highlighters

Activity

Active

- [ ] Walking [ ] Gym
- [ ] Housework [ ] Hydrotherapy

Passive

- [ ] Reading [ ] TV
- [ ] Music [ ] Light Housework

Meals

Breakfast

Lunch

Dinner

Snacks & Dessert

Beverages

- [ ] Juice [ ] Tea [ ] Water
- [ ] Milk [ ] Soft D [ ] Coffee
- [ ] Energy

Symptoms

Date: ____ / ____ / ____   Day ___

Sleep

	am / pm
Bed (last night)	_____
Asleep	_____ am / pm
Woke up	_____ am / pm
# of Disruptions	_____
Total Hours slept	_____

Medications

☐ No Change in Meds

☐ Dosage Changed

☐ New Medication

Details

Today's Ratings

Scale: 0 = None, 10 = Severe

Pain	_____ / 10
Fatigue	_____ / 10
Weakness	_____ / 10
Stiffness	_____ / 10
Anxiety	_____ / 10
Depression	_____ / 10
Stress	_____ / 10
Anger	_____ / 10
Brain Fog / Forgetfulness	_____ / 10

Pain location(s)

Circle or shade in where your pain is using pen, pencil or highlighters

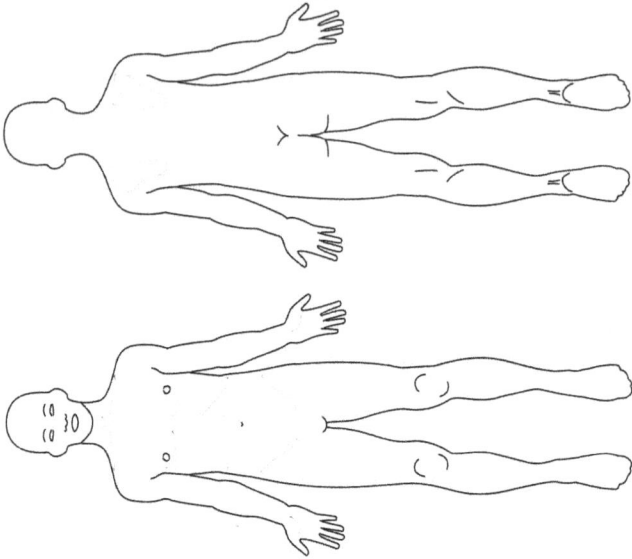

Symptoms

Meals

Breakfast

Lunch

Dinner

Snacks & Dessert

Beverages

☐ Juice ☐ Tea ☐ Water
☐ Milk ☐ Soft D ☐ Coffee
                   ☐ Energy

Activity

Active

☐ Walking ☐ Gym
☐ Housework ☐ Hydrotherapy

Passive

☐ Reading ☐ TV
☐ Music ☐ Light Housework

Date: ____ / ____ / ____   Day ____

Sleep

Bed (last night)   _____ am / pm

Asleep   _____ am / pm

Woke up   _____ am / pm

# of Disruptions   _____

Total Hours slept   _____

Medications

☐ No Change in Meds

☐ Dosage Changed

☐ New Medication

Details _____

_____

Today's Ratings
Scale: 0 = None, 10 = Severe

Pain   _____ / 10

Fatigue   _____ / 10

Weakness   _____ / 10

Stiffness   _____ / 10

Anxiety   _____ / 10

Depression   _____ / 10

Stress   _____ / 10

Anger   _____ / 10

Brain Fog /
Forgetfulness   _____ / 10

Pain location(s)

Circle or shade in where your pain is using pen, pencil or highlighters

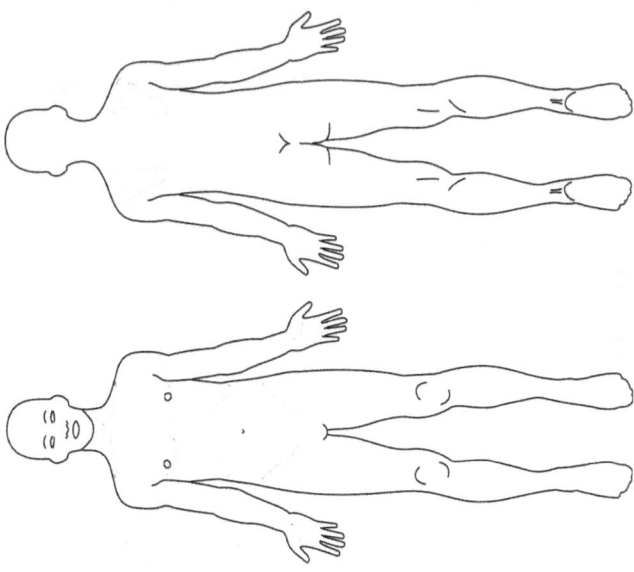

Symptoms

Meals

Breakfast

Lunch

Dinner

Snacks & Dessert

Beverages

☐ Juice ☐ Tea ☐ Water
☐ Milk ☐ Soft D ☐ Coffee
☐ Energy

Activity

Active

☐ Walking ☐ Gym
☐ Housework ☐ Hydrotherapy

Passive

☐ Reading ☐ TV
☐ Music ☐ Light Housework

Date: _____ / _____ / _____   Day _____

Sleep

Bed (last night)	_____	am / pm
Asleep	_____	am / pm
Woke up	_____	am / pm
# of Disruptions	_____	
Total Hours slept	_____	

Medications

☐ No Change in Meds
☐ Dosage Changed
☐ New Medication

Details _____

_____

Today's Ratings

Scale: 0 = None, 10 = Severe

Pain	_____ / 10
Fatigue	_____ / 10
Weakness	_____ / 10
Stiffness	_____ / 10
Anxiety	_____ / 10
Depression	_____ / 10
Stress	_____ / 10
Anger	_____ / 10
Brain Fog / Forgetfulness	_____ / 10

Pain location(s)

Circle or shade in where your pain is using pen, pencil or highlighters

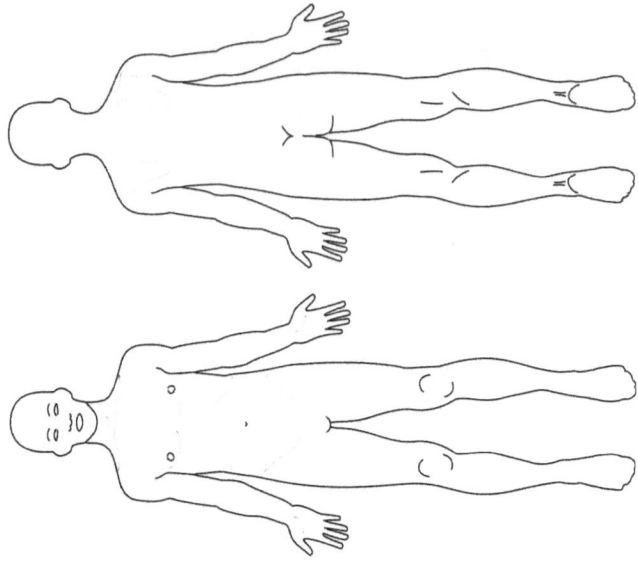

Symptoms

Meals

Breakfast

Lunch

Dinner

Snacks & Dessert

Beverages

- [ ] Juice
- [ ] Milk
- [ ] Tea
- [ ] Soft D
- [ ] Water
- [ ] Coffee
- [ ] Energy

Activity

Active

- [ ] Walking
- [ ] Housework
- [ ] Gym
- [ ] Hydrotherapy

Passive

- [ ] Reading
- [ ] Music
- [ ] TV
- [ ] Light Housework

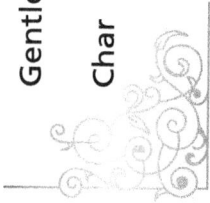

Dear User,

Thank you
for using this
Chronic Pain & Fatigue Diary!

I hope the information you recorded leads you to figuring out what triggers your pain level to flare up, and or this leads you to getting a diagnosis so you can get the proper treatment and support you need.

Gentle hugs!

Char

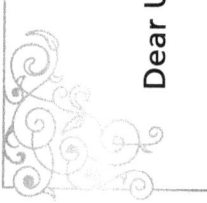